RATIONING SANITY

Hastings Center Studies in Ethics

A SERIES EDITED BY

Gregory Kaebnick and Daniel Callahan

This series of books, published by The Hastings Center and Georgetown University Press, examines ethical issues in medicine and the life sciences. Established in 1969, the Hastings Center, located in Garrison, New York, is an independent, nonprofit, and nonpartisan research organization. The work of the Center is mainly carried out through research projects, the publication of the *Hastings Center Report* and *IRB: A Review of Human Subjects Research*, and numerous workshops, conferences, lectures, and consultations. The *Hastings Center Studies in Ethics* series brings the ongoing research of The Hastings Center to a wider audience.

Contents

v

List of Figures

Acknowledgments

THANKS IN THE first instance must go to the participants of the project from which these essays grew and to the MacArthur Foundation for making the project possible. Philip Boyle, now vice president for ethics at the Catholic Health East Health System, formerly associate for medical ethics at The Hastings Center, did a great deal to prepare the material here for publication, and Ms. Lou Daniels, of the Center for the Study of Medical Ethics and Humanities at Duke University, was enormously helpful to me as I took over the task of seeing through the project to the end. Much of my work on *Rationing Sanity* took place during my year as a visiting scholar at Duke; I am deeply grateful to Jeremy Sugarman, then-director of the Duke Center, for arranging that delightful year. I also appreciate that Greg Kaebnick and his colleagues at Hastings thought of me when it came to finishing this job and that Richard Brown of Georgetown University Press was unfailingly patient. Thanks in the last instance are due to Hilde Lindemann Nelson, associate professor of philosophy at Michigan State, who always helps.

Introduction: Rationing Sanity

James Lindemann Nelson

ALTHOUGH SUFFERING FROM any kind of serious illness brings with it risks of stigma and (at least in countries such as the United States) impoverishment, people ill with a psychological or behavioral disorder suffer under a particularly dark cloud. To be—or to have been—mentally ill is still seen in many social contexts as *essentially* damaged, as defective in those features of cognition or agency that we tend to prize as distinctive to and definitive of human personhood. To face mental illness is to face problems that have been resistant to standard medical intervention and thus to rely on forms of care that may be either largely custodial in nature or on the fringe of the kind of substantiated scientific knowledge that (as many of us fondly imagine) characterizes health care generally considered. Even when what seem to be highly promising or effective therapies do appear—for example, in the case of depression or anxiety—by a curious inversion of the logic of stigmatization, even being *cured* can seem vaguely unsatisfactory. Shedding anxiety or depression under the influence of Paxil or Prozac strikes some as short-circuiting the "right" way for people to recover their psychological equilibrium: not by the exercise of will and thus as an expression of character, but rather via "merely" causal mechanisms.

These accompaniments of psychological illnesses—with the exception, perhaps, of scruples about *how* one is cured—have had a troublesome impact on the character of mental health insurance. Health care policies have traditionally made stark distinctions between the kind of underwriting they supply for "physical" ailments and that provided for mental illness, much to the disadvantage of the latter. From the perspective of publicly supported mental health care, deinstitutionalization, coupled with a lack of support for community-based mental health initiatives, has had highly visible consequences for many people suffering from severe and persistent psychological and behavioral problems.

Recently, debates about "parity" have been prominent, with Congress and the White House studying, considering, but—as of this writing—not enacting legislation that would mandate no invidious distinction between support for mental or physical health care by insurers. Yet an even more significant issue has been less a matter of media attention and public concern—the shift to using the tech-

1

niques of managed care to finance mental health services in both private and public settings.

Managed care as a strategy for funding health care has undergone such changes in recent years that there is even some controversy over whether it retains sufficient unity to be a useful focus of attention. But the effort to expose health care spending to the disciplines of the marketplace, in contrast to the "old days" of traditional indemnity insurance arrangements paying customary fees for services determined to be necessary by the very people who profited from them, remains vigorous. There's no room for complacency about whether patient welfare is being slighted in order to achieve economies.

This concern becomes more worrisome as mental health care becomes progressively further "managed." The traditional tendency to slight behavioral and emotional disorders—to see them as a mélange of the imaginary, the intractable, and the stigmatizing—depicts spending for mental health as a tub with a swift leak and thus spurs efforts to shut off the particular spigot that is filling it. Nor is there a large and effective constituency eager to monitor the performance of managed mental health care. Although there are surely well-organized groups such as the National Alliance for the Mentally Ill and the Barbizon Center for Mental Health Law serving as watchdogs, the drive to engage broad public concern in guaranteeing the quality of mental health care is blunted by the widespread and quite erroneous belief that mental illness is very rare and therefore not much of a threat to anyone not already ill.

And yet, it has to be acknowledged that concern about how much society and individuals allocate to the care of the mentally ill is not simply an obsession of morally dubious insurance executives trying to boost their bottom lines at the expense of the suffering. Health care spending in general absorbs an enormous and rapidly growing portion of the total economy, and those costs threaten society's ability to discharge other extremely significant responsibilities. Whether managed care is unfairly harming the ill is a very serious question. It should not, however, be confused with the concern that some ill people may not be as well off under the current regime as they might be under other imaginable ways of financing health care. The answer to this problem cannot be seen solely as a matter of providing ever more resources. The resources are limited; the needs, indefinitely great. The challenge is to determine what is fair.

As part of its ongoing efforts to contribute to fostering the best possible thinking on issues concerning the morality of our health care practices, The Hastings Center, with the generous support of the John D. and Catherine T. MacArthur Foundation, called together a collection of mental health care providers, scholars of mental health care, and bioethicists. This working group was charged with exploring some of the central regions of the large and contested terrain constituted by the use of managed care modalities to fund mental health care. The essays published here are part of the results of their research.

The joint work of these researchers took place in the mid-1990s, and several of the chapters of this book took their original shapes then. Although most have been reworked in the interim, responding to recent alterations in managed mental health's mise-en-scène, all the chapters address dimensions of the ethics of managed mental health care of persistent philosophical and practical urgency. Some offer answers to general questions about the kind of theoretical resources necessary to illuminate and resolve the issues. Others respond to a well known challenge to bioethics leveled by Norman Daniels. Daniels asked the field to answer four questions raised by any effort to justly ration health care: the question of how to balance everyone's claim to a "fair chance" at scarce resources with the value of maximizing the impact of those rare goods (the "best outcomes/fair chances" problem); the question of how much those who were worst off should be favored in the distribution of such goods (the priority problem); the question of whether and to what extent small benefits to many people should be allowed to outweigh great benefits to a few people (the aggregation problem); and the question of the extent to which decisions about the distribution of rare goods should be left to a representative, democratic process (the democracy problem).[1]

A distinctive feature of this collection is that answers to Daniels's questions are offered in the managed mental health context by some of the scholars who have been most prominently involved in approaching issues of rationing in this way, whereas others explore the extent to which the managed care context challenges the entire moral structure presupposed by the Daniels-inspired debate. At the same time, savvy clinicians continually assess the answers offered, examining the extent to which theoretical solutions make practical sense, offering their own distinctive perspectives on which avenues are most promising and which are most problematic.

Gary Belkin's chapter opens the collection, taking up the theme of managed care's impact on standards of clinical rationality, with special reference to mental health. He argues that the standard ethical analyses of managed care miss its most problematic features. Customary approaches to managed care assess it in terms of norms and analytical techniques developed by bioethicists in the 1960s and 1970s in response to a different set of challenges. By mistakenly thinking that those ideas are not conditioned by their historical context, bioethicists misunderstand both what made them originally persuasive and what has changed as we have moved into a time highly influenced by the presence of managed care. What is most important about managed care's influence is not fiscal, or even primarily ethical; the fundamental change that managed care introduces is epistemological. Our fundamental ideas of what constitutes valid medical knowledge are changing as a function of this change in medicine's fiscal structure.

Belkin further argues that the change in our understanding of medical knowledge is not innocent of power relationships and of cultural norms. "Evidence-based medicine" isn't merely a matter of developing techniques that reveal medical reality more thoroughly, more efficiently, and more usefully. Rather its dominance reflects a preference for the aggregate over the individual that is significantly influenced by powerful social interests.

Allen Buchanan's chapter might be seen as an instance of the kind of "normal bioethics" approach to managed care ethics of which Belkin is suspicious. In a thorough discussion of what constitutes practical rationality in professional management contexts, Buchanan argues that good managerial reasoning includes a significant role for ethical norms—at least in the sense that there is no necessary impediment to their influence. If we allow that excellence in service is included in the ethics of professional management, as Buchanan argues is the case, then there is no conflict of principle between physician ethics and managed care, because the challenge of a physician in managed care—to reconcile patient welfare with a fiscally responsible bottom line—simply is the challenge of professional ethics in competitive economic organizations.

Buchanan notes that the "fee-for-service" structure obscured how deep the doctors' commitment to patient welfare actually was, because it was set up in a way that aimed at their convergence. Managed care allows us to see how real that commitment is. This theme introduces the distinction between "status trust" and "merit trust." Status trust, an attribute of twentieth-century medicine, is enjoyed simply by virtue of holding a certain social role and is, as Buchanan sees it, highly suspect. Merit trust, in contrast, can be earned by doctors as individuals, depending on whether they achieve service excellence.

Buchanan's chapter can be seen as engaging with Belkin's critique to the extent that Buchanan makes a case that professional managers are not amoral maximizers of profit or even mere profit maximizers within legal and institutional constraints. What doctors may now be well advised to do is to turn to professional managers as canny guides to how the difficult virtue of excellence in service to consumers can be achieved within profit-driven systems. Although the need to pay closer attention to the epistemic implications of social shifts (and the social implications of epistemic shifts) remains, the sense that a managerial standard of rationality and knowledge must work to the detriment of ill people in particular, or the community in general, is made more problematic by Buchanan's argument.

Frances Kamm's chapter focuses on a particular antipsychotic drug, clozapine, as a case study of how to think about a rationing situation that cannot be altogether resolved by policy-level decisions that insulate providers from making crucial decisions about who should receive care and who should forego it. Clozapine is a drug to which different people will respond differently. Some will enjoy robust benefits, becoming so near to normal that they will be able to live independently, and even generate enough income to take over the fiscal responsibility for obtaining the drug. Others, unfortunately, will not be so lucky—they will benefit from the drug, but not sufficiently to live independently. Whether a given patient will be a "high" or only a moderate responder to the drug can only be determined after a trial of treatment.

Assuming that fiscal realities preclude providing clozapine to everyone who experiences any benefit from it at all, Kamm sees the moral problem here as whether those patients who achieve only moderate response—though still enjoying a kind of benefit that other medications may not be able to achieve for them—should forego further use of the drug so that the medication can be freed up for the use of others who might achieve a more substantial benefit and, at the same time, themselves take on the costs of their own care, allowing still others to benefit from the limited stocks available through public programs. Kamm exactingly lays out a number of morally pertinent considerations that reveal the complexity of questions of this sort, making plain how such considerations as need and urgency, time of treatment, and number treated make it ethically naïve to respond to such questions by merely looking to maximize good outcomes (or, for that matter, to rely on other simple principles, such as "it would always be wrong to discontinue a patient under treatment who was benefiting from the treatment").

Eric Rakowski returns to the level of policy, arguing for an approach that allows decision makers to sidestep the kinds of concerns that occupy Kamm and other philosophers who attempt to arrive at well-motivated answers to the problems that she and Daniels have articulated. Rather than worry about a morally authoritative answer to questions of aggregation, for example, or about how to most defensibly make trade-offs between fair chances and best outcomes, Rakowski argues that allocation should be determined by the insurance choices that people have made prior to developing a health need. Of course, not all have the ability to buy insurance, and some individuals—conspicuously including some people with mental illness, as well as children—have never been in a position to make prudent choices about what kind of health care they would elect. To cover instances of these sorts, Rakowski advocates a hypothetical form of reasoning. Rather than try to determine what morality demands, a proxy decision maker's job is to do her best to choose as the individual in question would have chosen for herself, had the possibility of choice presented itself. Although this is not a simple matter, it does not require solving difficult moral problems.

Several of the remaining chapters speak directly to Rakowski's approach. Bentson McFarland claims that the aggregation problem confronts clinicians working in managed care contexts daily. Patients with bipolar disorder, for example, sometimes require a great deal of a clinician's attention to achieve a therapeutic outcome that may be disappointingly meager. Time invested with such patients cannot be offered to patients with therapeutically more tractable conditions, such as anxiety or unipolar depression. To resolve this problem in a fashion that is maximally respectful of autonomy, as Rakowski suggests, would involve asking what insurance choices such people either did or would have made. As McFarland points out, however, there are serious complications to this approach if we acknowledge that some will choose not to insure adequately against illnesses or traumas they will suffer. If a society is not willing to simply allow such people who cannot afford out-of-pocket expenses to suffer without aid, then it will have to adopt what McFarland calls a "limited autonomy" model, in which a publicly funded "safety net" is established. This approach brings with it not only questions of moral hazard but also problems about the extent and form of funding—problems that include issues of aggregation, priority, and fair chances versus best outcomes.

Laura Weiss Roberts, Teresita McCarty, and Sally K. Severino examine Rakowski's position from another clinically sophisticated viewpoint. Their primary concern is that Rakowski's understanding of autonomy is too severely idealized to accommodate the actual situation of many mentally ill people and hence cannot successfully motivate an appropriate understanding of what justice demands for their care. In support of their criticism, Roberts, McCarty, and Severino draw heavily from empirical work on informed consent. They read this work as showing that making health care decisions in a way that fully expresses a person's autonomy requires repeated, clinician-guided explorations of options, risks, and potential benefits and note additionally that people's choices in hypothetical situations often differ from the decisions they make when confronted with a choice with real consequences. The unreliability of projection from hypothetical to real contexts seems pertinent to Rakowski's dependence on hypothetical projections as a way to deal with problematic cases in which individuals had no opportunity to make insurance choices, and the point that even mentally healthy people find the making of autonomous decisions concerning complex issues a chore raises further questions about the applicability of Rakowski's model to mental health care contexts.

Dan Brock's chapter addresses what seems to be a natural way of responding to the difficulties of fairly distributing mental health care. If we can't come to agreement on how much priority to give the worst off or on how we should rate the claim of best outcomes against the claim of fair chances or whether many small benefits can be measured against scarcer, more significant benefits, then we should rely on some kind of fair procedure—paradigmatically, on voting. Yet Brock shows how the resort to democratic procedures contains its own moral problems. The chief difficulty is not that the result of a vote may contradict what intuition or theory show to be more defensible resolutions of certain rationing problems—after all, we don't possess anything close to consensus about these matters—but rather that the result of voting per se can't be reasonably seen as a just resolution. Brock argues that any such votes would have to take place within a context of thoughtful deliberation, a deliberation that should aim to set the participants' values in a coherent, well-informed state. The decision makers ought not to see each other as merely trading off conflicting interests but as engaging in moral inquiry. Brock suggests that Charles Beitz's notion of "complex proceduralism" may provide for public deliberation the kind of justificatory force that the process of placing views in "wide reflective equilibrium" promises to achieve for individuals.

David Pollack discusses the experience of establishing health care priorities for Medicaid funding in Oregon in terms of the distinctions advanced in Brock's essay. In Pollack's view, those deliberations represented a substantial, good-faith effort to deliberate in a fashion that is tolerably close to the model Brock outlines. Pollack also provides a list of concerns that emerge from Oregon's complex and prolonged process that uncovers further, very practical problems, some of which hinge on such basic but crucial facts as that not all deliberators have the time or stamina to be effective in defending their conceptions of the best way to ration health care.

In my chapter, I explore to what extent those who are worst off can be said to deserve preferential allocation of resources. I consider challenges to a "preference for the worst off" principle that claim that it conflicts with sound theory (this includes joining in the discussion of Rakowski's work) before turning to the claims that it has counterintuitive implications and that it would have to be arbitrarily defined to do useful work. I end by defending a version of the worst-off principle that sees it as able to withstand theoretical challenges and as capable of being focused in a way that allows it to remain a useful contributor in our efforts to make rationing decisions fairly.

Tia Powell's concluding essay concretely addresses the ethical situation of the physician within managed mental health care. The hallmark of managed care is to constrain physician decision making in order to limit costs of care; the challenge is to define and navigate those constraints so that an acceptably high quality of care is maintained. To achieve this balance, Powell advocates an understanding of physician integrity within managed care that highlights three dimensions of duty. The first, cooperation, denotes the physician's responsibility to participate in the structuring of a reasonable standard of care for the plans they work with and to help managed care organizations realize in an effective way that general standards must be fit to the needs of individual patients. The second, appeal, refers to the duty of doctors to appeal unreasonable denials of reimbursement for care that they determine is medically necessary; Powell notes that an institutional context that made appeal less difficult and expensive for physicians would help contribute to faithful performance of this duty. The third, evaluation, is the doctor's duty to help the patient understand and assess such matters as the financial incentives that are operating in ways that may affect the physician's decisions.

A person dealing with mental illness is caught between a serious malady that often remains poorly understood by both caregivers and the community and a rapidly evolving health care structure still seeking an acceptable balance between patient welfare and fiscal solvency. As many of the chapters of this collection show, mediating this tension requires careful, philosophically sophisticated, clinically informed thinking. It also requires that professional caregivers show a kind of moral grit, as others of the chapters here attest. But every bit as fundamental, dealing justly with the claims of mentally ill people in a substantially reconfigured health care environment needs a wider moral discussion conducted by a society that is currently much preoccupied with other matters—a discussion in which people with firsthand experience of mental illness must play a very significant part. Many of the contributors to this volume have made substantial contributions toward getting these kinds of concerns more centrally on the social agenda; we all share the hope that this book will contribute to making the dialogue more richly thoughtful.

Note

1. Norman Daniels, "Four Unresolved Rationing Problems: A Challenge," *Hastings Center Report* 24, no. 4 (1994): 27–29.

CHAPTER 1

Shifting the Focus: The Historical Meaning of Managed Care and the Search for Ethics in Mental Health

Gary S. Belkin

THE PRIMARY ETHICAL challenge of managed care, in my view, is not how it is a bump in the road of work on justice, autonomy, community, or beneficence: that is, not in how it is a familiar bioethics problem with new details. If we approach the dilemmas that managed care raises as just another species of justice problem or autonomy problem, we do so at our peril. Indeed, perhaps we *always* approach the myriad of dilemmas that fall under the hegemony of bioethics discourse for their solution and understanding with a stock menu of overarching concepts ("autonomy," "justice," "competence," etc.) at our peril. Use of these tools risks wielding a cookie-cutter approach that obscures other socially and historically contingent patterns and relevant factors that shape what is experienced as the "ethical."

In the case of managed care, such quickness to apply familiar terms and analysis ignored its central feature: its rewriting of what counts as medical knowledge and the critical role of accepted versions of what counts as relevant medical knowledge in lending coherence to ethical terms in the first place. The ethics of managed mental health care is a particularly powerful example of this. In perhaps no other area of medicine have conflicts about how to go about validating facts and knowledge or establishing how disease is proven and known been so explicitly contested. Managed care's ethical uniqueness is not how it tweaks old concepts but how it reflects and permits the stealth infusion of a new epistemology for certifying factual knowledge in medicine. Use of the same old ethical analyses deployed in the last decade missed how they were hostage to, and inadequate to engage, this larger historical challenge.

Justice Theory and Autonomy Digest Managed Care: Who Was Eating Whom?

The bioethics industry began to set is sights on managed care in the early to mid-1990s. For one thing, their focus seemed to vindicate and further generate a literature that saw medical ethics as primarily an encounter with problems of justice theory. "Medical ethics," wrote Ezekiel J. Emanuel, "must stop being case oriented and become institutionally oriented. We bioethicists must stop approaching problems from a philosophical perspective and adopt a political science perspective. Nothing makes this more clear than the challenges of managed care. Traditionally, medical ethics has focused on cases and the ethical issues that arise between individual physicians and patients. . . . By contrast, medical ethics has not been as successful . . . in problems that involve the healthcare system. This is probably most clear in the rather disappointing contribution medical ethics has made to the problem of allocating health care resources."[1]

Emanuel was in the forefront of an effort to reconfigure ethical problems of health care as distributive conflicts around health care resources and as the result of failed or poorly considered political structures. As he argued in his earlier book *The Ends of Human Life*, "It is the failure of political philosophy that underlies the contemporary deliberations in medical ethics, of liberalism, to provide such guidance that has created the current preoccupation with and irresolution of medical ethical questions."[2] That effort to cast what had often been discussed as interpersonal duties and expectations between doctors and patients as instead structures of public deliberation and distribution seemed a growing part of the bioethics literature at the time.[3] For Emanuel and others, managed care vindicated the wisdom of their focus on the prominence of such political institutional issues in bioethics. It was an approach congruent with the conviction of managed care's advocates that the appearance of managed care was an inevitable response to insufficient efforts, if not a crisis in efforts, to set limits to health care expenditures and rationally distribute medical resources. Yet even granting such a crisis, justice theory advocates within bioethics, by quickly seeing in managed care validation of their own agenda, limited what could be said about managed care. Managed care and ethics in that analysis validated one another, but by skipping an important step. There was limited analysis as to the source within managed care of their common assumption that certain problems in the health care system were best managed and characterized as institutionally remediable.

The old bioethical discourse accommodated the new. Attempts were made to cast consumer insurance choice itself as the autonomy that patients prized within the discipline.[4] Eric Rakowski, for example, argued that many of our concerns about which claims by patients on their physicians or on society have moral weight become unproblematic if we reexamine our understanding of the nature of patient autonomy. Insurance plans that set limits on care were indeed picked and deliberated upon by individual, autonomous, respected agents exercising their choice. The need to mediate who deserved what kind of access to medical care or to establish how individual benefits from treatment were compared and prioritized vanishes when individuals' "preferences as insurance buyers, not the morality of their actions . . . determine what care they receive. . . . The allocation of health care ought to depend entirely on which precautions people have freely chosen to invest in. . . . [I]n a just world private insurance is best seen as an autonomy-respecting substitute for the more comprehensive insurance against misfortune that justice otherwise mandates."[5] Efforts such as these to adopt revised meanings to older terms risked employing terminology that lost its prior meaning but that invoked its old authority, becoming MacIntyrean "fragments," where we talk as if its original meaning and value remained true.[6] By this process managed care was positioned, to its ultimate benefit, within legitimate approaches to bioethics.

Of course, many refused to recast a commitment to autonomy principlism as compatible, if not rejuvenated, with managed care. The characterization of patients as respected and fundamental arbiters of their best interests at each point of medical decision making remained a strongly advocated position that found, in managed care, practices inimical to patient autonomy.[7] Others advanced what I would call a "middle position." From this middle position some sought to embrace the need for "systemwide reform" but to also "be careful to preserve what is most valuable within [the physician ethics] tradition."[8] It recognized the impossibility of unrestrained physician advocacy and patient autonomy and the need to systematically discipline the system so it could affordably meet the needs of all citizens, but it sought as well to preserve the centrality of private physician-doctor decision making to the idea of ethical medical practice:

> If parties other than the physician and patient determine what treatment is necessary and appropriate for an individual patient, the therapeutic relationship will be so severely eroded as to render it meaningless and ineffective. This does not mean that physician practices cannot or should not be monitored or that issues of cost are irrelevant, but it highlights the importance of taking decisions about rationing and the appropriateness of care out of the consultation room and away from the bedside and bringing these debates to the level of the conference table and the community.[9]

Here is an example of confidence that the rules of managed care could be written in such a way as to permit physician-patient dyads to flourish.[10] Somehow these tensions could be in balance, and the chairman of the AMA's Council of Ethical and Judicial Affairs could assert that "the value both of justice and individualism" can be realized and "a physician's obligation to society must complement his or her obligation to provide individual patient care."[11] Even avowed critics of doctor-patient focused ethics who pursued the alternative of political theory did not seem able to escape this paralyzing dichotomy.[12] The "middle road" hoped to hold on to and thus reconcile principled commitment to a just process of shared deliberation with individual prerogative and choice.

But autonomy-revisionist, autonomy-preservationist, and middle-road views shared a great deal. They all reflected efforts to reckon with the implications of new institutions shaping medical practices and the asserted relevance of an ethical point of view that addressed corporate and political behavior.[13] More importantly, though, in their differences over how to reckon with these challenges, they generally shared assumptions about the nature of medical knowledge. Bioethics took shape several decades ago to highlight the moral transactions at stake in individual doctor-patient encounters, to identify moral elements and implications of doctors' knowledge in doctor visits. It presumed and used a picture of medical knowledge as something accessible to individuals and understood in the context of their needs but drawn from a pool of clinically derived, expert-sanctioned knowledge and scientific laboratory investigation. Problems of covenants, contracts, beneficence, and even justice all generally began at a similar place regarding what kind of thing medical knowledge was.[14] Managed care rested, however, in a very different place, fundamentally challenging what medical practice and medical knowledge was. The "we told you so" chorus from the now de-marginalized interest in justice and political theory as bioethical theory only dimly perceived and made explicit the implications of really taking on such a reconfiguration of medical knowledge. Autonomy critiques as well as endorsements of managed care, preoccupied with extending meanings and agendas meant for old targets to new ones, missed what was changing in the process, changes particularly consequential for mental health care.

The "Real" Managed Care Stands Up: Managed Care as a Technology, and the Ethics of Measured Experience

Critics of medical technology assessment have argued that ethical analysis merely evaluates the impact—but shares and leaves behind unquestioned the rationales and imperatives—of the appearance of technologies themselves.[15] Ethical approaches to managed care may have similarly traveled the same terrain as ethical analysis, but these approaches left their features poorly mapped. Technology assessment can risk taking on only the "effects" of a technology, thus seeing it as extrinsic to the interests and contingencies of the social world. Ethical assessment similarly missed the depth of social constructedness and the nature of powerful social change and interests that converged in the most challenging aspect of managed care—a new paradigm of medical knowledge. This needed to be the more direct focus of ethical inquiry. Redefining managed care as a justice problem or shoehorning it as a familiar autonomy problem avoided contending with the ethical and existential challenges that result from defining the experience of an impaired individual through summation of the experience of many others.

The analogy with technology assessment is apt. Managed care explicitly represented itself as a new technology. It offered measures of medical work and effectiveness far more rational and reliable than physician judgment could provide, and it drew upon the rhetoric and aspirations of health services researchers and their asserted ability to know more than individual physicians could know by looking at aggregate data. John Wennberg, for example, clearly asserted that he offered a distinct science that revealed and corrected the more limited focus of "biomedical science":

The role of biomedical science is to generate ideas and technologies; it is the role of the evaluative sciences to provide the necessary clinical information linking treatment to outcomes. But the evaluative sciences are neglected.[16]

To address this neglect, Wennberg pursued federal sponsorship of health services research and is credited with the creation of Agency for Health Care Policy and Research (now the Agency for Healthcare Research and Quality— AHCPR). This event was seen as the triumph of a new science, a new way to explain and understand disease:

The law's passage also represented an important step in the evolution of medical decision making. With growing rapidity in the 1970s and 1980s, patient care decisions moved from the domain of the treating physician (perhaps in conjunction with the patient) to being the domain of objective knowledge, and from a matter of great subjectivity ('clinical judgment') to a matter of such objectivity that patient care decisions could be reviewed and affirmed or denied by individuals who did not even see the patient.[17]

Medical discourse was to be replaced with measurable items in order to create what Paul Ellwood envisioned as "a new universal language to communicate hurting, functioning, working, interacting, and living."[18]

Rather than an inevitable response to cost control and economic inefficiency, managed care is more plausibly placed within a history of appeals to standardized and ostensibly objective measures and models of human behavior to resolve contentious issues in complex and modern capitalist democratic societies. Briefly put, what was, and is, up for grabs is not simply an autonomy model versus a communitarian model or a physician-virtue account or a program of just distributive structures. Similarly, what is particularly unique about managed care is not its threat to autonomy or its possibilities for community or its incompatibility with physician values or its logical response to resource constraints per se. What is primarily up for grabs—and cuts across as well as is shaped by these other questions—is how we will recognize valid medical knowledge. Managed care's success in furthering certain social interests was accomplished through a particular transformation in how we speak knowledgeably about medical things. In this case, the 1960s' and 1970s' battles over whether what doctors and patients did when they met would be talked about in clinical or in philosophical terms are not as relevant. The more pressing challenge is whether we will talk about medicine in terms of if its practitioners' practices and skills contain the knowledge they need for clinical decision making or whether valid medical knowledge is better known from aggregated experiences of individuals outside of any particular encounter. It is a question of epistemically privileging standardized information over judgment, of quantified measurement over experience. Such a contest has a long history and invites careful examination of its ethical costs and benefits.

Managed care was not an inevitable solution to the real challenges of cost containment. But it was an understandable, if not predictable, turn given historical scholarship that sees resolution of policy disputes accomplished frequently, and perhaps increasingly, by transforming them into problems of measurement. Managed care needs to be understood as a potentially radical transformation in the epistemology of illness and treatment. Its claim to objectivity and standard measurement fits in a long line of attempts to satisfy wishes for open, reliable, presumably nonsubjective methods to resolve controversy by changing a question of expert judgment to one of technical formula. It similarly fits into a history of employing aggregate measures and standardized products and processes to mobilize and deploy (though not necessarily to conserve) large amounts of capital. Managed care is one of many examples in which far-reaching changes in political economy were facilitated by replacing knowledge generated and confirmed in face-to-face experience or by expert judgment with standardized information shared by anonymous individuals often at a distance from each other.

Expansion of markets, for example, required reliable knowledge of product quality, in large numbers, over large distances, sight unseen. Trusted practices arose as proxies for what had been direct experience, and their use, in turn, created its own validating framework. Once grain quality—or, for that matter, cell lines or patient symptoms—were codified in such a system of measurement, that codification shaped grain prices, experimental practice, and pathological phenomena whose experienced reliability in the context of that system confirmed the very logic of the classificatory or measuring system.[19] If one can devise criteria for three grades of grain to characterize the infinite variation provided by nature, then one can trade and price at a distance by using such averaged measures without requiring on-site inspection directly by buyers. The criteria then take on an inevitability and correctness. Standardized quantification has often been critical to developing such "technologies of trust," which then permitted the complex practices of industrialized societies.[20] Averaged outcomes from a particular therapeutic intervention and its protocol project a uniform patient experience that allows both predictable resource use when such intervention is provided to a large population and a way to implement uniform action by multiple individuals using shared methods of performance evaluation. From CPR to chemotherapy protocols, the mass distribution of medical therapy has, before managed care and like so many sectors of our private and public life, capitalized on the power of conceiving and creating the subject as an aggregate.[21] The epistemic problem of managed care summing experience to determine medical truth and reality is no different from grain grading in that it is a convenience to enable certain kinds of exchange and scale of distribution and confidence in that distribution. It was not the only way to distribute medical resources, nor the only "scientific" way.

Advocates of managed mental health care conceded as much when discussing the importance of standardized diagnostic systems:

> Our [view] . . . does not rest on a view of disease and disability as ultimately real in a metaphysical sense. . . . Society, however, needs a publicly acceptable and administrable system for defining boundaries of health insurance coverage. The conception of mental disorders embodied in DSM-IV provides a workable definition of those boundaries.[22]

A consequence of making treatment rules or judging the relative value of interventions based on averaged experience is that subsequently established practices may *make* experience confirm the logic of the practice:

> If 80 percent of all patients with a given condition inevitably die, and if this figure is used to make normative decisions to forego care on a particular patient, then his/her death is entered into the next statistical base, rendering it more likely that an ever increasing number of patients who are faced with the same condition will die, thus creating self-fulfilling and circular arguments.[23]

What are the ethical implications of conforming individual experience to an average? Is there an ethical distinction between locating authority over decisions about managing one's body in individual experts and locating it in shared rules of decision making? Does it make an ethical difference whether we expose persons to the judgment of individual uncertain knowledge or to collectively approved certainty? How are epistemologies of fact and ethics linked?

Knowledge and Power in Managed Mental Health Care

This mutually reinforcing relationship between conventions of organizing knowledge and social interests in pursuing certain forms of clinical practices was particularly manifest in managed mental health care. Mental health is an area of medicine where clashes over explanatory paradigms of disease can be particularly explicit. The very notion of what it means to say that a mental illness is a disease has undergone marked change in the last several decades. The significant revision a quarter century ago in the Diagnostic and Statistical Manual (DSM) system of mental health diagnosis reflected a deliberate effort to adopt a nosology that ostensibly avoided commitment to a particular theory or etiologic system but that would be based simply upon reported or demonstrated symptom clusters that were easily verifiable and resistant to wide subjective interpretation. Following the symptom menu, different clinicians should arrive at similar results.

This change was asserted to be a more scientific step, offering objective agreement where individual subjectivity dispersed any hope of manipulatable measurable categories. However, such a change in the DSM, from DSM-II to DSM-III, was pursued by a minority within the American Psychiatric Association who saw a psychiatry based upon social, experiential, and developmental frameworks of mental illness and treatment as unscientific because they were prone to subjective, nonverifiable "abuse." The ease and perceived unruliness with which a range of behaviors could be considered pathological ran into the antipsychiatry movement. It also began to worry government officials in the mid-1970s, at a time of newly constricted funding for mental health services that left insurers starting to feel the runaway nature of costs. With optimism about national health insurance, psychiatry did not want to be left out. The emerging growth and interest in larger-scale clinical trials research also required a reliable tool with which diagnosis held some trusted, standard meaning. Papers in the psychiatry literature had noted the problem of poor diagnostic reliability since the 1940s, but the premier value of reliability—the identification of standardized reliability as a (if not *the*) difficulty facing psychiatry— required the set of social, political, and cultural circumstances that came together in the 1970s.[24]

The context within which DSM-III appeared to be logical and compelling is forgotten, and only its logic and compulsion remain, assisted by a self-referential validating body of research data and experience. Rather than one of a range of possible systems organizing clinical experience and adopted in response to a complex set of social factors, the DSM regime has assumed unique authority. It is not unearned. Dividing the world in the way it does enabled and enhanced a shared conversation—people could agree on what they were saying when using a diagnostic term. Doing so also permitted measuring the impact of certain interventions and generalizing such findings. But the efficacy of such findings is by definition then known only within and among those same categories. Nature offers many connections and fruitful interventions betwixt and between categories we may have made up for reasons having much less to do with any "natural" order of things than with a social one.[25] The ways we arrange meaningful data and agree on its relevance do not satisfy any less cultural imperatives, because they successfully predict things we do to (our) nature. We can divide the world up in ways driven very much by reasons of culture and still get results. The value of the so-called postmodern critique of science is not that a scientific finding is a mirage but that it is a selective picture chosen for many reasons other than purely "natural" ones and one that can quickly assume authority and exclusivity as an account of nature as long as it permits enough social interests to work. The history of science is filled with powerful examples of the self-fulfilling prophecy whereby technique maps nature in its own image.[26]

So, genetic variation by diagnosis or differential response to certain drugs could be found in nosological systems other than DSM,[27] and valid clinical knowledge is often found outside such systems altogether.[28] The important question is how did what is now understood as a scientific classification become the compelling paradigm? In the context of managed mental health care, this is a significant question. A nosology that was chosen for its emphasis on manifestation over cause and agreement and generalizability over individual impression, judgment, or subjective experience was in retrospect a prized tool for managed care's ascendancy, dovetailing neatly with efforts to transform and commodify mental health experience as a strategy for containing it. This facilitated the ability of managed care efforts to be seen as part of a logical, scientific transformation. And that connection, critical to the success of managed care, recast how mental health professionals understood themselves. Short-term treatments, particularly those based in cognitive behavioral theory and traditions focusing on discrete measurable outcomes and behaviors, were suddenly written in as scientifically "getting the last word," as "right all along" compared to their more costly, less standardizable, introspective, psychotherapeutic competitors.

DSM permitted confidence in a managed claim of distanced and standardized certainty about patient experience and appropriate care. The apparent objectivity and reality of the diagnostic scheme provided confidence in managed care's authority to reliably distinguish between what was "necessary" care and what was not. James E. Sabin and Norman Daniels confidently argued that

the model prescribes compassion for those who are less fortunate in the natural lottery that distributes capabilities, but makes the health sector responsible for correcting only those conditions which—in DSM-IV terms—can be diagnosed as . . . mental disorders. . . . The normal function model holds that health care insurance coverage should be restricted to disadvantages caused by disease and disability unless society explicitly decides to use it to mitigate other forms of disadvantage as well.[29]

This importance of diagnosis in guiding managed care's categorization of necessity was disputed. William Glazer, for example, argued that custodial and necessary care could be indistinguishable in mental health and that standard measures of function and impairment were more important than the presence or absence of disease.[30] These positions, however, were united by a shared confidence in standardized measuring, further confirming this as a key change enabling a managed care regime. The prominence of this shift in focus is further underscored by comparison with 1970s concerns over precisely the same issues of custodial versus medically necessary functions of psychiatric work—concerns in which this interest in and confident reliance upon aggregate measuring or outcomes scoring were totally absent.[31]

"Setting formal priorities requires a continuous mechanism for identification and evaluation of health measurement and outcome data. . . . [P]riorities should be set by a mechanism that is accountable, enhances objectivity, and allows for a public participatory process."[32] This widely read endorsement of the ability of managed care to set priorities for mental health interventions, avoiding allegedly "ideological" whims of prior mental health reform cycles, was ironically accomplished by not questioning the ideology present in the new face of justice theory advocated here—a confidence in certain measures tempered by public deliberation over the menu of measuring tools and decision trees.

Attribution of objectivity to outcome measures is not a technical feat, it is a cultural accomplishment. It is not "common sense" but the result of commodifying medical exchange so that it is amenable to new ways of manipulation and accessible to new corporate and public authority. The determination that such practices are "better" reflects culture, not just science. The scientific crutch offered new power that public deliberative ethics otherwise lacked. It was not the inevitable pathway for incorporating such theory into bioethics. By taking the pathway of outcomes measurements bioethics joined managed care, however critical of its "effects," in a less-examined commitment to a world of medicine by aggregate measure. This can result in the benefit or detriment of doctors and patients. The point I am making here is that bioethics should be aware of the norms that it often implicitly accepts (as it did/does with doctor-patient–centered medical knowledge) and also pose ethical questions about the underlying changes that have reoriented presumed norms. Without doing so, revised autonomy accounts and enthusiastic justice theory on the one hand and physician-virtue ethics or persistent individual inviolable autonomy accounts on the other simply navigated, and continue to navigate, between the rock of apology and the hard place of irrelevance.

Take, for example, the assertions and criticisms behind Philip J. Boyle and Daniel Callahan's prominent discussion of managed mental health care.[33] These authors argued that criticism of managed mental health care was often overblown and tied to those whose interests were threatened, and its ethics needed to be placed in the light of the fee-for-service alternative. Managed care could further ethically laudable gains where fee-for-service failed, such as in expanding access. Boyle and Callahan openly embraced the knowledge assumptions of managed mental health care but did not see how that move shaped their ethical assessment, rather than vice versa. The asserted need for managed mental health organizations to know confidential medical information, for example, was simply assumed: How else could care be managed? "What is morally relevant is not whether managed mental health care plans need to know (they do), but rather how they will use and protect this information."[34] The ethical question was redefined as an issue of use (how will the accessed information be handled), rather than access (who has claim to access such information about other persons), not by ethical argument but by institutional imperative: managed care *needs* it to accomplish other goals. But this was an imperative based on subscribing to the epistemological assumptions of the managed care world and the new network of power and interests that facilitated, and was facilitated by, that worldview in force throughout the 1990s. Advocates of mental health services were hampered by "a relative lack of proof of the effectiveness of mental health treatments. . . . The lack of agreement regarding effectiveness gives rise to conflict even among mental health advocates."[35] Managed care offers clarity to such empirical dispute. However, this is not a moral position. It reflects cultural choice about using certain methods to resolve disagreement. Recall Sabin and Daniels's acknowledgment, quoted earlier, of DSM-IV as a practical tool for achieving consensus.

Even if managed care could not pin down the "elusive understanding of quality and uncertainty," the ideal that it could possibly do so defined the ethical standard. "The justification for fewer services grows stronger in the absence of a good definition of quality," especially for less severe illness.[36] Because such proof may be hard to come by, these authors argued, there then exists an ethical continuum of obligations depending on the efficacy data available. To call this continuum moral is, however, to conflate a moral value system with a measuring one, or to at least admit that ethical norms are pliable, contingent, and shaped by premises about specific measurement techniques. Similarly, to assert that "medical professionals may be expert in providing medical criteria, but they are not experts in what society prefers"—that being left to public discussion of "what is necessary and what kind of effectiveness is sought"[37]—seems to give lie to the firm, unbiased nature of such outcomes data and their unique contributions to forms of deliberation over health care. To argue that "the rise of managed mental health organization shows clearly that much of the moral debate has been misfocused" on "the individual patient and physician . . . completely neglect[ing] the social fabric"[38] was historical tautology. The rise of managed care should be explored directly not inferentially through its consistency with a preferred, unrelated agenda. What *had* changed was that a new medical episte-mology favoring certain social interests gave traditions of justice theory, institu-tional ethics, and the like an air of inevitability and correctness.

The criticism aimed at Boyle and Callahan's argument, when it appeared, underscores this reading. Within that criticism, what distinguished those who attempted to justify managed mental health as ethical and those who questioned such a connection were often differences over the epistemological shift at the heart of the managed care revolution. Mark Schlesinger urged caution as to what data could offer and how they are selectively used, thus seeing these authors as "masking a predisposition toward resource-conserving reforms in the guise of logical argument and empirical documentation."[39] Richard Surles criti-cized them for just the opposite—not pushing the agenda far enough to refocus what is of ethical importance in "considerations such as informed consumer choice of health care plans and the responsibility that those managers of those plans have in responding to requests for assistance." Predictably this shift in focus was underscored with a belief that managed behavioral health care was a "specialized technological innovation composed of sets of carefully planned protocols, which blend advanced information technology with clinical decision-making systems."[40]

Looking Back

Such "advanced-technological" aspirations have not materialized. Since the flurry of interest in joining bioethics and managed care briefly characterized here, managed care as a practice has both succeeded and failed. A new class of political interest groups and industry lobbying clout has emerged to assert and protect the ability of payers to set standards of medical necessity and enforce upon providers protocols and standards ostensibly reflecting sound, efficacious, and cost-effective medical practices. Most Americans receive their health care within a system of managed care. However, as of this writing, a brief dip in health expenditures of several years ago has been erased with insurance rate increases well into the double-digits and enough dissatisfaction with impedi-ments to care that many state legislatures have incorporated into statute their own conclusions about medical necessity, such as requiring coverage for extended maternity stays. A contentious debate over a federal "Patient's Bill of Rights" reflected the stalemate between the power and allure of market rational-ity that managed care has established on the one hand and the antipathy and public outrage that has, albeit variably, appeared in organized political action on the other. Managed care has not succeeded, but its logic and its institutions persist and seem firmly entrenched for the time being. The long-term planning and intense level of consumer education needed to make this market vision of a smart health care system work gave way to short-term cost-saving strategies, encouraging everyone, including providers, to become short-term schemers not "advanced clinical decision mak[ers]." Increasing volume and creatively offering services—rather than expanding quality, educating patients, or investing the time and energy to promote healthy lifestyles—have been the only real incentives that managed care has offered providers. Although there are indications that eclectic quality assessment may emerge as a gatekeeper for reimbursement (as opposed to, for example, concrete utilization targets), success in such efforts will require rethinking the assumptions about economic incentives and population-based interventions underlying managed care and its critique of individual judgment.[41]

Managed care has not yet proven to be a source of sweeping change in rationalizing the system or providing nascent structures for community participation in shaping a just process of rationing and resource utilization. It has primarily accomplished a huge transfer of income from providers to managers and successfully advanced a discourse of market behavior of which we can't seem to get out but also from which we have not clearly gotten much in return. Enthusiasm for standardized measures in clinical practice and for gold standards of clinical science has accelerated beyond the initial facilitative role the legitimacy that such efforts had in the confidence that payers could "manage" treatment decisions. That enthusiasm has particularly taken hold of the mental health field. But I predict that the faith in such research, protocols, and standards to guide appropriate treatment will also disappoint; there have been indications of a possible critical response to their scientific authority.[42] Such methods often do not clarify how and when variation in outcome reflects characteristics of patients—rather than therapies or provider skills. Aggregate measures can only ask certain research questions, which are not always reflective of the main choices and dilemmas facing clinical practice. They also have marginalized complex psychological skills and experience to the long-term detriment and potential irrelevance of a distinct psychiatric profession.

DSM has reflected and furthered an altered culture of knowledge production, within which managed care has thrived, such that superficial summary statements can correlate with standardized goals that enable management of large populations, the predictability and reliability of response at a population level, and the ability to command large amounts of capital. The generalizability of normed measures, the assumption that practice variation reflects poor quality, and the standardization of outcome as the goal of managing systems of care are practices that still present both unclear policy gains in proportion to the enthusiasm they generated and ethical questions that have yet to be squarely faced.

Managed care and the practice of evidence-based medicine resonate with a much larger phenomenon—the accelerating use of appeals to standardized measures and a historically select notion of scientific authority to resolve politically contentious issues—what I have elsewhere called the "technocratic wish."[43] Medicine is relatively new to these issues. The industry is beginning to prefer routine and abstracted measures over the individualized history and pathology that dominated medical practice around the turn of the twentieth century. Whether these changes will lead to a new structure of medical rationality and consideration of the medically and mentally ill subject in ways that promote welfare, well-being, equitable and efficient use of our common resources, and the further advancement of knowledge toward those ends remains to be seen. However, barring creative leadership from the new managing elite, the prognosis for such success is not good.

Whatever the turn of events, bioethics needs to return to its earliest stated aspiration: the critical analysis of efforts to reduce the suffering individual to scientific constructions, be they physiologic or economic ones. Bioethical inquiry needs to be more curious about the historical moment in which it finds itself. The challenges and questions raised by the fragmentation of the medical subject and its re-creation as an economic actor or an average probability may require broad reconsideration of the bioethical toolkit and point to new intellectual touchstones and traditions— Foucault instead of Kant, history and sociology of science instead of philosophy, Habermas instead of Rawls. The early response to managed care illustrates the distance that bioethics needs to go to move from being a newly entrenched profession to a mature scholarly discipline.

Notes

Author's Note: Several years have passed since the original preparation of this chapter for a volume inspired by a series of Hastings Center–sponsored meetings in 1995 and 1996. It captured a pressing preoccupation of a group of bioethicists at the time: Was managed care—in particular managed mental health care—ethical? Did it provide an opportunity to realize procedural justice and judicious resource use, or did it instead violate principles of autonomy? Asked to revise that chapter for this publication, I decided to keep it generally intact but to introduce generous new use of the past tense. From the perspective of this writing it seems helpful to revisit for its own sake that early- to mid-1990s discussion. Although subsequent attention has been somewhat less preoccupying and pressing, the issues from that slice in time that I emphasize here endure and offer useful insights into the evolution of the medical marketplace and its ethics.

At that time, as now, I was concerned that the attention given to managed care by bioethicists risked shielding both managed care and bioethics from scrutiny of their own histories. The attempt to equate familiar ethical paradigms with managed care challenges missed the important ways, for example, managed care "rationing" was quite different from prior circumstances in which an "equity" vocabulary had been deployed to assess it. I urged caution about the degree to which managed care absorbed the projections of our premanaged care concerns or worldviews. The ease with which managed care was translated as a "justice problem" or an "autonomy problem" tied it to particular idioms and analytic purposes too quickly. Such translations may have represented it in unique ways that were more familiarly digestible but not necessarily in ways that were, or are, the most perceptive or useful.

1. Ezekiel J. Emanuel, "Medical Ethics in the Era of Managed Care: The Need for Institutional Structures Instead of Principles for Individual Cases," *Journal of Clinical Ethics* 6, no. 4 (1995): 335–38, 335. This particular issue of the journal captured the literature and concerns of the time and is used illustratively here.

2. Ezekiel J. Emanuel, *The Ends of Human Life* (Cambridge, Mass.: Harvard University Press, 1991), 13. Emanuel's work was a widely read attempt to further a central role for justice and political theory in bioethics that was part of a miniwave of such interest, building on the work of others, although with somewhat different targets. See, for example, Norman Daniels, *Just Health Care* (New York: Cambridge University Press, 1991); and A. Troyen Brennan, *Just Doctoring: Medical Ethics in the Liberal State* (Berkeley: University of California Press, 1991).

3. For example, discussions of futility and necessity of medical interventions, often viewed through notions of physician fidelity and responsibilities, were recast by some as problems of this sort. See Daniel Callahan, "Medical Futility, Medical Necessity—The-Problem-Without-a-Name," *Hastings Center Report* 21, no. 4 (July–August 1991): 3–35. Or see Norman Daniels's discussion of cost-containment policy as a question of liberalism in "Why Saying No to Patients in the United States Is So Hard," *New England Journal of Medicine* 314, no. 21 (1986): 1380–83. See also Steven H. Miles and Robert Koepp, "Comments on the AMA Report 'Ethical Issues in Managed Care,'" *Journal of Clinical Ethics* 6, no. 4 (1995): 306–11. For further consideration by Emanuel of the possibilities of managed care organizations serving as a framework for political determinations by communities of health care priorities, see Ezekiel J. Emanuel and Linda L. Emanuel, "Preserving Community in Health Care," *Journal of Health Politics, Policy, and Law* 22, no. 1 (1997): 147–84.

4. E. Haavi Morreim, *Balancing Act* (Boston: Kluwer Academic Publishers, 1991); for Eric Rakowski's discussion of just allocation of mental health care, see chapter 4 of this book.

5. See Rakowski, chapter 4 of this book.

6. Alasdair MacIntyre, *After Virtue* (Notre Dame, Ind.: University of Notre Dame Press, 1981). The value here of MacIntyre's widely quoted book is not its focus on the fate and significance of virtue-ethics but on a more underlying assumption about philosophy as a historical process—that changes in theory need to be understood not as ideas set independently on their own footing but as specific responses and adaptations to what preceded them.

7. Typical examples include Daniel Sulmasy, "Managed Care and the New Medical Paternalism," *Journal of Clinical Ethics* 6, no. 4 (1995): 324–26; Frank A. Chervanak and Laurence B. McCullogh, "The Threat of the New Managed Care Practice of Medicine to Patient's Autonomy," *Journal of Clinical Ethics* 6, no. 4 (1995): 320–23.

8. Susan M. Wolf, "Health Care Reform and the Future of Physician Ethics," *Hastings Center Report* 24, no. 2 (March–April 1994): 28–40, 28, 34.

9. Alan R. Fleischman, "Physicians and Ethics in the Health Care Reform Debate," *Hastings Center Report* 24, no. 3 (May–June 1994): 10–11.

10. Wolf, "Health Care Reform." For the specific case of balancing commutative and distributive obligations, with the nod toward the former in cases of conflict, see Edmund Pellegrino, "Interests, Obligations and Justice: Some Notes toward an Ethic of Managed Care," *Journal of Clinical Ethics* 6, no. 4 (1995): 312–17.

11. Charles W. Plows, "A Response to Comments on the AMA Report 'Ethical Issues in Managed Care,'" *Journal of Clinical Ethics* 6, no. 4 (1995): 318–19, 319.

12. For example, Emanuel, after asserting a need to depart from doctor-patient case ethics, continued to argue how "we have been rather poor at elucidating the type of institutional arrangements that affect fulfillment of the requirement of informed consent or confidentiality in individual cases. This focus on ethical principles and rules is no longer tenable—if it ever was" (Emanuel, "Medical Ethics," 335). Such a focus may be "untenable," but it is in this passage precisely what the "institutional arrangements" are meant to preserve. Elsewhere, Emanuel offered a core notion of the doctor-patient relationship that was threatened and deserved to be preserved. Ezekiel J. Emanuel and Nancy Neveloff Dubler, "Preserving the Physician-Patient Relationship in the Era of Managed Care," *JAMA* 273, no. 4 (1995): 323–29. If political arrangements are merely a house to secure other ethical notions, than what does it mean to assert them as critical in explaining and surmounting medical ethical dilemmas? What is happening in this part of ethics—that speaks of rules structuring society and its largesse—to make its disbursement just, but whose faith in such rules is belied by a wish that they somehow will permit, if not privilege, a core process of individuals relating? How comfortable is communitarianism with relying upon community?

13. This included the argument revisited earlier not only that performing as an economic actor in the market lent ethical value and autonomy but conversely that corporate business entities carried the same obligations that had usually been given to individual doctors acting with and for their patients. For Allen Buchanan's discussion of the ethics of managed care, see chapter 2 of this book.

14. Rarely are these assumptions explicitly discussed in the way in which I am concerned here. An important and illustrative exception is H. Tristram Engelhardt's *The Foundations of Bioethics* (New York: Oxford University Press, 1986). Here he explicitly explored the historical contingency and social construction of diagnosis to support a notion of secular autonomy and patient-centered authority. Although I argue elsewhere that this and other bioethicists' use of historical interpretation is only selectively used, the point is that versions of medical knowledge are intimately tied to versions of ethical justification in medicine. Engelhardt's apparent rejection of physician categories still located the debate within the context of these doctor-patient

encounters and remained in an ethical world concerned with individual treatment decisions, of what doctors owe specific patients and what they can come to know together. Managed care challenged the relevance of that point of view. For advocacy of the necessity of more sophisticated historical contextual understanding of the emergence and use of bioethical thinking and practice in order to keep bioethics useful and relevant, see Gary S. Belkin, "Toward a Historical Ethics," *Cambridge Quarterly of Healthcare Ethics* 10 (2001): 345–50, and Gary S. Belkin and Allan Brandt, "Bioethics: Using Its Historical and Social Context," *International Anesthesiology Clinics* 39, no. 3 (summer 2001): 1–11.

15. Henk M. J. ten Have, "Medical Technology Assessment and Ethics," *Hastings Center Report* 25, no. 5 (September–October 1995): 13–19.

16. John Wennberg, "AHCPR and the Strategy for Health Care Reform," *Health Affairs* 11 (winter 1992): 67–71, 67.

17. Bradford Gray, "The Legislative Battle over Health Services Research," *Health Affairs* 11 (winter 1992): 38–66, 64. Outcomes measures are frequently referred to as a new "technology" distinct from medical technology. Indeed, much of the literature is preoccupied more with what it takes to sell the technology rather than whether it is of any value. One study explored in obsessive detail the aspects of an automated health questionnaire that served to make it friendly to patients, convenient to use, and accepted by physicians in their offices. The fact that the device and its evaluation of health status were identical to that determined independently by the physicians studied received little comment. See Michael Roizen et al., "Can Patients Use an Automated Questionnaire to Define Their Current Health Status?" *Medical Care* 30, no. 5, supplement (May 1992): 74–84. For a critique during this period of the claim to science by health services researchers that resonates with much of the analysis offered here, see David Frankford, "Scientism and Economism in the Regulation of Health Care," *Journal of Health Politics, Policy, and Law* 19, no. 4 (1992): 773–99.

18. Paul Ellwood, "Shattuck Lecture—Outcomes Management: A Technology of Patient Experience," *New England Journal of Medicine* 318, no. 23 (June 1988): 1549–56, 1551.

19. Ilana Lowy and Jean Paul Gaudilliere, "Disciplining Cancer: Mice and the Practice of Genetic Purity," unpublished manuscript, and Ilana Lowy, "Tissue Groups and Cadaver Kidney Sharing: Sociocultural Aspects of Medical Controversy," *International Journal of Technology Assessment in Health Care* 2 (1986): 195–218. In these articles, the authors provide compelling examples of how social and cultural factors influence how and if clinical and experimental practices adopt standardized, homogenized industrial practices and methods or more localized, variable, craft knowledge and individualized decision making. In terms of patient symptoms, how the DSM is a perfect example of this facilitative standardization and made mental health care particularly vulnerable to managed care is discussed further later.

20. Theodore Porter, *Trust in Numbers* (Princeton, N.J.: Princeton University Press, 1995). For the development of the grain market, see William Cronon, *Nature's Metropolis: Chicago and the Great West* (New York: Norton, 1991), and how it is discussed in Porter, *Trust in Numbers*, 46–48.

21. Stefan Timmermans and Marc Berg, "Standardization in Action: Achieving Local Universality through Medical Protocols," *Social Studies of Science* 27 (1997): 273–305.

22. James E. Sabin and Norman Daniels, "Determining 'Medical Necessity' in Mental Health Practice," *Hastings Center Report* 24, no. 6 (November–December 1994): 5–13, 12.

23. Laurie Zoloth-Dorfman and Susan Rubin, "The Patient as a Commodity: Managed Care and the Question of Ethics," *Journal of Clinical Ethics* 7, no. 4 (1996): 339–57, 350.

24. Mitchell Wilson, "DSM-III and the Transformation of American Psychiatry: A History," *American Journal of Psychiatry* 150, no. 3 (March 1993): 399–410.

25. I do not want to exaggerate this distinction between the "social" and the "natural." Indeed, the approach to the sociology of scientific knowledge I subscribe to here precisely underscores how these categories remake each other yet also retain some distinctiveness. Helpful sources that capture the range of work contributing to this approach include Andrew Pickering, *The Mangle of Practice—Time, Agency, and Science* (Chicago: University of Chicago Press, 1995); and John V. Pickstone, *Ways of Knowing: A New History of Science, Technology, and Medicine* (Chicago: University of Chicago Press, 2001).

26. For example, with regard to topics in mental health, see Kurt Danzinger, *Constructing the Subject: Historical Origins of Psychological Research* (New York: Cambridge University Press, 1990); Ian Hacking, *Rewriting the Soul: Multiple Personality and the Sciences of Memory* (Princeton, N.J.: Princeton University Press, 1995); David Healy, *The Anti-Depressant Era* (Cambridge, Mass.: Harvard University Press, 1997).

27. Charles G. Costello, "Research on Symptoms Versus Research on Syndromes—Arguments in Favor of Allocating More Research Time to the Study of Symptoms," *British Journal of Psychiatry* 160 (1992): 304–8.

28. R. H. Cawley, "Psychiatry Is More Than a Science," *British Journal of Psychiatry* 162 (1993): 154–60.

29. Sabin and Daniels, "Determining 'Medical Necessity,'" 10.

30. William M. Glazer, "Psychiatry and Medical Necessity," *Psychiatric Annals* 22, no. 7 (July 1992): 362–66.

31. Boris M. Astrachan, Daniel J. Levinson, and David A. Adler, "The Impact of National Health Insurance on the Tasks and Practice of Psychiatry," *Archives of General Psychiatry* 33 (July 1976): 785–94.

32. Philip J. Boyle and Daniel Callahan, "Minds and Hearts: Priorities in Mental Health Services," *Hastings Center Report* 93 special supplement (September–October 1993): 21.

33. Philip J. Boyle and Daniel Callahan, "Managed Care in Mental Health: The Ethical Issues," *Health Affairs* 14, no. 3 (1995): 7–22.

34. Ibid., 16.

35. Ibid., 10.

36. Ibid., 13.

37. Ibid., 19.

38. Ibid., 20.

39. Mark Schlesinger, "Ethical Issues in Policy Advocacy," *Health Affairs* 14, no. 3 (1995): 23–29, 23.

40. Richard Surles, "Broadening the Ethical Analysis of Managed Care," *Health Affairs* 14, no. 3 (1995): 29–31, 30.

41. Although I do not have the space to elaborate on this point, I find public health models of prevention and intervention to be quite distinct in their regard for the subject and their assumptions about the relationship between aggregate and individual experience from the commodification, manipulation, and homogenization at the core of assumptions undergirding both managed care and simplified routines of driving practice through standardized categories and algorithms.

42. D. D. R. Williams and Jane Garner, "The Case against 'The Evidence': A Different Perspective on Evidence-Based Medicine," *British Journal of Psychiatry* 180 (January 2002): 8–12.

43. Gary S. Belkin, "The Technocratic Wish: Making Sense and Finding Power in the Managed Medical Marketplace," *Journal of Health Politics, Policy, and Law* 22, no. 2 (1997): 509–32.

CHAPTER 2

The Ethics of Managed Care:
Medical Ethics or Business Ethics?

Allen Buchanan

NO ONE DENIES that the growth of managed care poses ethical problems. The fear most often voiced is that physicians will be subject to pressures to limit utilization in order to reduce costs and that quality of care will suffer. There is disagreement, however, about whether managed care presents novel ethical problems and about whether the realities of managed care are compatible with the ethical practice of medicine.

Some ways of describing the shift to managed care beg questions concerning these disagreements. For example, if the advent of managed care is described as the transition from medicine as a profession to health care as a mere business or as the change from a patient-centered activity to a profit-maximizing activity, then we are already well on our way to concluding that managed care presents wholly novel ethical issues and that managed care and medical ethics are incompatible.

To avoid such question begging, I will begin with what I hope will be a neutral and accurate description of the shift to managed care. By managed care I shall mean, as a first approximation, efforts to control costs in the provision of health care by controlling utilization through techniques such as the following:

1. Requiring preauthorization for certain services and procedures (e.g., hospital admission)
2. Using primary care physicians as gatekeepers who control patients' access to specialists
3. Payment limits on types of services in publicly funded programs (such as Diagnostic Related Groups [DRGs] in Medicare hospital reimbursement)
4. Various arrangments designed to give physicians financial incentives to limit utilization of care (including profit sharing through limited partnerships with hospitals, physician compensation based on capitation, various forms of financial risk–sharing with physicians such as making

year-end bonuses or the return to physicians of "holdbacks" from rev-
enues contingent on the meeting of individual or group targets for limiting utilization)

Though it points us in the right direction, such a definition is inadequate. It
fails to capture explicitly a feature that proves crucial for understanding the
ethics of managed care: the fact that these techniques for limiting utilization
are, for the most part, developed and administered by persons steeped in the
culture and ethos of organizations, and of organizations of a particular sort,
namely, business organizations in which managerial professionalism—which
should be distinguished from medical professionalism (as it has hitherto
existed)—dominates.

For this reason I will characterize the current revolution in health care, the
shift to managed care, as a transition from a system in which care was generally
provided by physicians who were relatively independent of organizational constraints and in which medical professionalism was dominant to a system in
which physicians are significantly subject to organizational constraints and in
which medical professionalism is to a substantial degree subordinated to managerial professionalism.

This way of describing the transition to managed care enables us to frame the
ethical issues in a fruitful way. First, we can articulate the ethics of organizations—in particular, of organizations in which managerial professionals dominate. What is meant here by "ethics" is normative ethics: we are inquiring into
what sort of conduct individuals within such organizations ought to follow.
Next, we can inquire as to whether the (normative) ethics of these sorts of
organizations can or cannot accommodate what is most valuable in medical
ethics, in particular, a commitment to the patient's welfare and a respect for the
autonomy of competent patients. Finally, if it turns out that there is no incompatibility, then we can move on to the next crucial question: Under what conditions is it reasonable to expect an acceptable degree of compliance with sound
ethical principles within managed care organizations?

The ambitions of this article are modest. Here I only attempt to traverse the
first two steps—to articulate the ethics of the general type of organization of
which managed care organizations are instances and then to determine whether
this ethics can accommodate what we value most in medical ethics. No attempt
will be made here to lay out an account of the conditions that would facilitate
good compliance with the ethical principles in question.

To tackle the first stage of the inquiry, we must begin with an adequate characterization of the ethics of organizations in which managerial professionals are
dominant. Such organizations may be called bureaucratic organizations.

The phrase "bureaucratic organizations" is chosen to convey breadth—to
include organizations that may not qualify as bureaucracies strictly speaking but

that are sufficiently like the paradigm cases of bureaucracies that an ethical analysis that applies to the latter will illuminate them as well. Bureaucratic organizations have the following features:

1. Personnel are arranged in a hierarchy of authority (though there are some nonhierarchical, that is, equal status or authority, relationships as well).
2. There is a complex division of labor with an array of distinct roles (positions), each understood as having a sphere of authorized action, where the assignment of individuals to particular roles is understood to be based, at least in principle, upon merit earned through the appropriate exercise of expertise.
3. Those occupying policy making or higher-level administrative positions in these organizations identify themselves and are generally regarded by others as professional managers (or professional administrators).
4. Many if not most of the products or services ("outputs") of the organization are either joint or collective—produced by the cooperation of a number of individuals and subgroups.
5. The day-to-day practices and decision-making procedures of such organizations rely heavily on rules and policies that are typically recorded in written form.
6. To a large extent, the roles that individuals occupy in such organizations can be explained in terms of principal-agent relationships.

This characterization seems to satisfy the requirement of breadth: it applies to government bureaucracies, for-profit corporate bureaucracies, and not-for-profit bureaucracies.

The third and sixth features in particular warrant expansion and are intimately related through the concept of managerial professionalism. Included in the concept of managerial professionalism are several ideas: (a) that professionals are an elite whose status is based on excellence in the exercise of special expertise; (b) that the expertise qualifies as a form of practical rationality, understood as including the use of various techniques of rational decision making based on more or less formal calculations of costs and benefits or on the ranking of alternatives according to articulated technical criteria; and (c) that, as a professional, the individual is understood to be an agent acting for various principals and as the bearer of their trust, where this trust is based upon either belief in the agent's skills and commitment to excellence or upon the reputation of the organization, or both.

Two types of principals may be distinguished: external and internal. In the case of for-profit corporate bureaucracies, the stockholders are the chief external principals. In the case of government bureaucracies, the chief external principal is the general public (or some specified segment of it, as with government bureaucracies that serve certain limited constituencies, such as the Veterans' Administration). Internal principals are the individuals or groups within bureaucracies whose subordinates serve as their agents, acting ultimately on the bureaucracy's authority. Typically persons in such organizations operate as principals to some individuals in the organization (usually their subordinates) and as agents to others (usually their superiors). Often an individual serves as the agent of two or more principals. To the extent that the roles individuals occupy in bureaucracies can be explained in terms of principal-agent relationships, we can think of bureaucratic organizations as webs of principal-agent relationships. Some threads of the web connect to points within the organization, some to points outside it.

The Ethics of Bureaucratic Organizations

For our purposes, the ethics of bureaucratic organizations are constituted by the following obligations or commitments that persons working within such organizations have, whether they adequately comply with them or not:

1. Organizational role-derived obligations and contractual obligations.
2. Extraorganizational general and special obligations.
3. Obligations that are responses to the agency risks inherent in bureaucratic organizations.
4. Obligations of corporate and collegial loyalty and of dissent (what might be called the ethics of "exit, voice, and loyalty," to borrow from Albert Hirschman's book of that title).
5. Commitments to excellence.

Role-Derived Obligations and Contractual Obligations

Most discussions of the ethics of organizations focus primarily, if not exclusively, on obligations derived from organizational roles and the conflicts that can arise between them and extraorganizational obligations. In these discussions the content of role-derived obligations is understood in a purely instrumental way, as being determined ultimately by the goals of the organization (or of its chief principals), as these are to be achieved through the division of labor among roles within the organization.

If we assume that the individual's taking on the organizational role is voluntary and that the organization's defining goals are morally legitimate, then the individual who assumes such a role has an ethical obligation to fulfill the particular duties attached to them. Assuming an organizational role is understood to have the moral effect of a promise to perform the tasks assigned to that role. So, under these conditions, role-derived obligations become ethical obligations. Similarly, in the performance of one's organizational role, one can incur contractual obligations. Just as one's role-derived obligations become ethical obligations, so do the contractual obligations one incurs in the performance of one's role.

However, obligations derived from organizational roles and contractual obligations are not absolute: they are limited by one's antecedent extraorganizational general and special obligations. And some of the most difficult problems of ethics for persons in bureaucratic organizations arise when there is a conflict between their role-derived obligations or contractual obligations, on the one hand, and their extraorganizational obligations, whether special or general, on the other.

Extraorganizational Special and General Obligations

An individual's extraorganizational special obligations to her family or friends or to persons generally can sometimes conflict with the obligations of her organizational role. In some cases, what will be required to resolve the conflict will be a balancing of obligations, preferably by appeal to a higher-order principle that establishes priorities among them. The results of such a balancing or prioritizing process may be difficult to predict in advance of actually having gone through it, in the richness of the concrete context in which the choice must be made. In general, however, this much can be said: the obligations that one freely assumes in becoming the agent of another or in taking on an organizational role do not absolve one of one's most important general obligations to others, especially those obligations that correspond to their rights as persons.

Obligations That Are Responses to the Agency Risks Inherent in Bureaucratic Organizations

The next element of the ethics of bureaucratic organizations is less obvious or familiar than the first three, but it is extremely important. The key idea is this: some of the most important ethical obligations of individuals in bureaucratic organizations are commitments that serve to reduce certain agency risks that result from the distinctive characteristics of these types of organization.

In any principal-agent relationship there are agency risks, risks that the behavior of the agent imposes on the principal, due to the fact that the agent may be in a position to pursue interests other than those of the principal at the principal's expense. Because of their distinctive features, bureaucratic organizations pose certain distinctive agency risks. Such risks can be reduced through regulation (with a system of rewards and punishments); through the terms of employment contracts; or by the inculcation of internal constraints, that is, by ethical commitments on the part of the agents who might otherwise impose the risks, or a combination of two or more of these three types of strategies.

Some agency risks, and hence some of the obligations of bureaucratic ethics that are responses to them, are common to a number of other principal-agent relationships (such as that between lawyer and client or financial advisor and client) that often do not exist within an organizational context. Other agency risks are peculiar to bureaucratic organizations because they arise from the distinctive features of such organizations—in particular, their hierarchical character and the fact that most products are jointly produced through a complex division of labor among experts.

The fact that some obligations are role derived is not distinctive of bureaucratic ethics, because nonbureaucratic organizations, as well as groups such as families, feature role-derived obligations as well. What is distinctive of bureaucratic ethics is best understood as being a response to the agency risks that are both inherent in this type of organization and peculiar to it.

I observed earlier that in the case of bureaucratic organizations there are both internal and external principals. For simplicity, and because it is most relevant to the concerns of this article, I will focus here on the risks that bureaucratic behavior poses for external principals, taking as paradigms the risks to shareholders of private corporations and the risks to the public in government organizations.

Among the most significant risks that bureaucratic behavior imposes on external principals are the following:

1. Inefficient use of resources—due to sheer waste, to failure to use the least costly effective means for achieving ends, and to diversion of resources to purchase unnecessary perquisites for bureaucrats or for hiring unnecessary personnel.
2. Outright misappropriation of resources—embezzlement; fraudulent requests for reimbursement for travel, equipment, and other expenses; as well as diversion of resources from projects for which they were intended to other legitimate projects.
3. Goal-substitution—cases in which bureaucrats covertly pursue their own goals (which may not be self-regarding) or those of other principals, rather than those of their authorized principals, in effect making and pursuing different policies under the guise of implementing authorized policies.
4. Passive opposition to directives or policies—by stalling on implementation, requesting further studies, more data, and so on as a deliberate though unacknowledged attempt to impede implementation.

5. Shirking—substituting leisure or the pursuit of unauthorized activities for compensated work time.
6. Expertise imperialism—representing tasks that do not fall within the agent's domain of expertise as doing so, in order to appropriate these activities or the resources available for pursuing them.
7. Partiality—basing rewards, personnel placement decisions, and advancement decisions on personal loyalties or extraorganizational allegiances, rather than on performance.

Again, note that some of these risks are not peculiar to bureaucratic organizations. For example, shirking is a risk in many if not all principal-agent relationships. Even so, the risk may be greater in bureaucratic organizations for a number of reasons. For example, when the division of labor is complex and particular roles involve the exercise of highly technical skills, shirking may be more difficult to detect. Similarly, where large amounts of money are involved and where the processes by which resources are allocated are extremely complex and involve actions by a large number of people over a considerable stretch of time, it may be easier to disguise misappropriations. Passive opposition may be easier to achieve without detection and hence less likely to be deterred by fear of punishment in a complex organization (some of whose inner workings are opaque, not only to external principals but also to many within the organization as well).

Some of the most central principles of bureaucratic ethics respond directly to the foregoing risks. For example, the fundamental tenet that bureaucrats are fiduciaries, entrusted with resources that belong to others (the principle of stewardship), is intended to express and to foster an ethical commitment, an internal constraint, to counter pressures of self-interest or extraorganizational allegiances that can lead to the inefficient use of organizational resources or to outright misappropriation. The intent of the ethical injunction expressed in the principle of stewardship is to impress upon the bureaucrat (or manager) that the resources she controls are not her property but rather are owned by others for whom she serves as trustee or steward.

The equally fundamental principle that bureaucrats are to observe the distinction between being an administrator and being a policymaker (the principle of the separation of powers) is an explicit response to the risk of goal-substitution. Although this principle does not provide a formula for determining when the boundary between implementation and policy making has been transgressed, it emphasizes that there must be such a boundary and that it must be respected.

Another of the central tenets of the ethics of bureaucratic organizations is the meritocratic principle. This principle is distinctive of bureaucratic organizations as opposed to organizations based on patronage or hereditary privilege and differentiates the bureaucratic organization as a modern phenomenon from its medieval and ancient predecessors, at least in the West. The meritocratic principle holds that selection of personnel for official positions should be based on merit, that performance of persons in the organization should be impartially evaluated according to task-related criteria, and that continued employment and advancement should depend upon excellence demonstrated by such impartial and appropriate evaluation. The commitment that this principle expresses is a direct response to the problems of passive opposition, shirking, and partiality.

For reasons that will soon become clear, the agency risks listed earlier, to which the preceding principles of the ethics of bureaucratic organizations are responses, may be called first-order agency risks. Analogously, the principles of obligation that express internal constraints designed to reduce these first-order risks may be called first-order obligations.

There are at least three all-too-familiar types of behavior often engaged in by those in bureaucratic organizations that thwart efforts to reduce first-order agency risks. Each of them has the function of making it difficult to detect behavior that puts principals at risk or to assign responsibility for undesirable actions or outcomes. Each type of behavior makes it hard to determine whether agents are acting in ways that create first-order risks and hence whether they are complying with the preceding (first-order) principles of obligation.

Behavior that fosters lack of accountability regarding first-order risks and compliance with first-order obligations may be characterized as follows:

1. Appeal to authority ("I was just following orders").
2. Failure to document activities and decisions in such a way as to make accurate evaluation of outcomes and assignment of responsibility possible.
3. Failure to specify duties or tasks concretely and to assign them unambiguously to particular agents or groups of agents.

Corresponding to these second-order agency risks are second-order obligations. These are principles that express ethical commitments, internal constraints whose function it is to reduce second-order risks to minimize the occurrence of the sorts of behaviors which, by undermining the conditions for accountability, make it difficult to determine whether first-order obligations are being fulfilled. For this reason, these second-order obligations may be referred to collectively under the label "obligations to ensure accountability." Among the most important of these are the following:

1. The obligation to ensure that there are clear lines of authority and responsibility—to see to it that individuals' roles in the organization and their attendant duties are specified concretely and consis-

tently (so far as this is possible without impairing needed flexibility and creativity).
2. The obligation to ensure that performance is monitored and evaluated adequately and that good performance is rewarded and poor performance corrected or penalized.
3. The obligation to provide adequate documentation.

When Bureaucratic Virtues Become Bureaucratic Vices

The preceding principles most clearly illustrate the main thesis of this approach to the ethics of bureaucratic organizations, namely, that the distinctive principles of bureaucratic ethics express internal constraints, ethical commitments that function to reduce the most serious agency risks inherent in bureaucratic organizations. At this point, however, a word of caution is in order. Ethical principles, or rather the commitments they express, are only one way of reducing agency risks. Ethics, as a variety of internal constraint, is to be contrasted with external incentives and regulations, whether positive (rewards) or negative (penalties), which are designed to reduce agency risks by achieving a closer congruence of the interests of agents and principals. In some cases, perhaps most clearly when the personal costs of honoring ethical commitments are extraordinarily high, appropriate incentives may be essential. In many cases, the best arrangement is to reinforce ethical commitments by rewarding ethical behavior and penalizing unethical behavior. In other words, the choice is rarely "ethics or incentives."

Ethical commitments do enjoy one signal advantage over externally imposed rewards and penalties: they avoid the costs of monitoring by third parties. The individual's own conscience serves to monitor his behavior (a "regulator" who follows him no matter where he goes), and the costs of monitoring are shifted from the organization to the individual. These are clearly advantages from the standpoint of the organization and the principals it serves.

Nevertheless, reliance on ethical commitments as opposed to incentives has its own costs. That this is so in the case of bureaucratic organizations becomes evident if one reflects upon the fact that bureaucratic virtues, if taken to extremes, become bureaucratic vices. For what I have referred to thus far as ethical commitments are—in an earlier vocabulary that has only recently begun to be resuscitated—virtues.

Virtues, roughly characterized, are commendable dispositions to act, to decide, to judge in certain ways, and to have certain sentiments in response to various situations. One of the chief virtues of bureaucrats is impartiality. Part of what it is to possess the virtue of impartiality is to have internalized the commitment expressed in the meritocratic principle discussed earlier and to apply that principle consistently. In the context of the managerial professionalism characteristic of bureaucratic organization, this means to a large extent the impartial application of criteria for evaluation that purchase quantification at the price of a high degree of standardization and abstraction. But as all of us who have dealt with bureaucracies (and who beyond the age of infancy in modern life has not?) know, impartiality can degenerate into an unthinking rigidity, a callous formalism that is blind to relevant differences among individual cases and puts too much stock in narrow quantification and calculation. Thus among the risks of reliance on ethical commitments—on virtues—as a way of reducing certain agency risks is the danger that other agency risks will be created if the disposition that the individual internalizes fails to include sufficient subtlety of judgment. For this reason, any serious consideration of the ethics of bureaucratic organizations, including managed care organizations, must recognize the need for developing processes of selection, training, and acculturation that foster and sustain good judgment. And here it is worth noting that one of the chief complaints of many physicians about managed care is that too often practice guidelines or other utilization criteria are applied rigidly, without proper appreciation for the nuances of particular cases.

Obligations of Loyalty and Dissent

The most familiar (because it is the most dramatic) example of this category of obligations is the obligation of whistle-blowing. In some cases, the individual working within an organization faces a conflict between either her own role-derived obligations or the organization's general policies on the one hand, and her general obligations to prevent harm to innocent persons or to prevent the misuse of citizens' or stockholders' resources on the other. But in other cases, the individual may be confronted with a conflict between her obligations to carry out her superior's directives and what she understands to be the commitments and goals of the organization. In either case, the individual may be obligated to attempt to change the policy or the directive and, failing that, even to refuse to comply with it. In some instances, if the harm to be averted is serious enough, the individual may be obligated to go outside the organization to the legal authorities or to the press in order to avoid serious harm.

The exact nature and extent of obligations of conscientious dissent, refusal, and disclosure (whistle-blowing) are complicated by two distinct factors. On the one hand, in some cases one's obligations are affected by the degree of risk to oneself (or one's family) that fulfilling them would entail. On the other, the trust that one's colleagues and superiors come to have in one, one's tacit and express commitments to the good of the organization, as well as one's obligations to minimize harm to innocent individuals (such as stockholders) must all be taken into account, if not in deciding whether to dissent or to blow the whistle, at least in a responsible determination of the manner and timing of doing so.

The ethics of dissent thus includes not only obligations to dissent but also obligations of responsible dissent.

The Commitment to Excellence

It is useful to list the commitment to excellence as a distinct component of the ethics of bureaucratic organizations for this reason: even if the formal definition of the individual's role in the organization specifies that she is responsible for excellence in the performance of this or that task, the commitment to excellence has at least two other sources as well. First, in well-functioning organizations, the organizational culture fosters and expects a commitment to excellence in the provision of products and services. (This may or may not be explicitly expressed in the corporation's mission statement.) Second, the individual's identity as a managerial professional includes a commitment to excellence that he or she brings to the role and that exists independently of the individual's allegiance to a particular corporation's mission statement.

To take only one example out of the many that are documented in the business ethics literature of the link between professionalism and the commitment to excellence, consider the case of an individual who resigns because the actual role assigned to him within the organization is incompatible with the commitment to being an excellent aeronautical engineer that led him to choose to work for this particular company in the first place. Here the individual experienced a profound disillusionment because the corporation misrepresented itself as having the same commitment to excellence that he, as a professional, espoused. To summarize, an individual's commitment to excellence is typically both a matter of her integrity (a commitment to her better self, as it were) and a commitment to others, so far as the individual represents herself as a person who is committed to excellence or pledges herself to further the goals of an organization whose culture includes a commitment to excellence.

As we shall see, one mistake commonly made by those who warn that managed care will convert medical professionals into mere businesspeople is the wholly unwarranted assumption that businesspeople as such have no commitment to excellence—that is, they care about the quality of their products and services only insofar as such quality contributes to maximizing profits for their organization or financial gain and advancement for themselves. What this assumption amounts to is a failure to see that there are professionals other than medical professionals (or that managerial professionals are among them). It is also a failure to see that as a matter of organizational culture or policy, as part of the definition of one's organizational role or as an element of a personal commitment so basic as to be a core element of one's professional identity, the commitment to excellence can provide a significant constraint on the pursuit of profit and on the strategy of merely responding to the wants or preferences of clients or consumers as distinct from their needs. Indeed, a failure to acknowledge the role of the commitment to excellence in business generally, and in the ethics of managerial professionals in particular, results in blindness to one of the basic ethical tasks of conscientious persons in bureaucratic organizations that operate in a competitive environment: the attempt to provide the best product or service for one's clients or customers while at the same time achieving an acceptable bottom line. To a large extent, excellence for managerial professionals is today commonly understood as the ability to achieve a high degree of congruence between these two commitments.

Furthermore, it would be a mistake to assume that whenever it is not possible to achieve congruence, in order to reconcile the commitment to providing the best product or services with an acceptable bottom line, the bottom line must take precedence. Whatever the extent of compliance with the ideal, managerial professionalism as a normative concept includes a refusal to participate in the provision of goods or services that fall below a minimum standard of quality.

Appreciating this fact about the ethics of bureaucratic organizations is important, because it shows quite clearly that there is nothing unique about the position of the conscientious physician (or other health care professional) who works in a managed care setting, at least so far as the general structure of ethical obligations is concerned. It is a truncated and distorted conception of organizations operating in a competitive environment that reduces their ethics to the pursuit of profit through role-derived obligations, bounded only by external, extraorganizational obligations.

It is therefore simply false to depict the physician (or other health care professional) as an alien being thrown into an amoral corporate culture. Instead, at a general level of description, the physician or other health care provider in the managed care setting faces precisely the same task that all managerial professionals face: reconciling the bottom line with their commitment to excellence, as a matter of individual professional identity and as a matter of role-responsibility or corporate culture and mission.

There are, of course, two features of health care that are especially significant, though not necessarily unique. First, because sometimes persons' lives literally may depend on the outcome of a given decision, the stakes may be higher more frequently in health care, including managed care, than in other competitive organizations. Second, in some cases, patients may be especially vulnerable in their interactions with physicians—or with other health care professionals, including nurses—because those interactions disclose intimate facts about the patient and revolve around some of life's most profound events and transitions. Nevertheless, even if it is true that high stakes and extreme vulnerability are more frequent in medical practice (or certain types of medical practice), it would be a mistake to assume that they are not present in the practice of other professionals. To cite only a few examples: structural engineers frequently make decisions upon which the lives of large numbers of individuals depend, investment specialists influence decisions that can have profound effects on a person's material well-being, and lawyers often are privy to the most intimate facts during a time of extreme personal crisis for their clients. The case of legal professionals is especially illustrative. Lawyers working in large law firms have always been faced with essentially the same ethical challenge that physicians in managed care organizations now face—how to reconcile the demands of their roles in competitive organizations subject to stringent financial cost-accounting with loyalty to their clients.

Managers and physicians in managed care organizations confront the same basic ethical task: providing the best care for patients compatible with an acceptable bottom line. Nevertheless, there is an ambiguity that must be explored more carefully in the notion of the commitment to excellence as it applies to managerial professionals. In laying out the distinctive features of bureaucratic organizations, I suggested that the normative conception of a professional manager or administrator within a bureaucratic organization of any kind includes the idea of a commitment to excellence in the performance of the distinctive activity of persons in such roles. That distinctive activity was seen to consist largely in the application of various more or less formalized techniques of practical rationality to decisions about the organization of production and personnel. Such techniques include highly quantitative methods of cost-benefit and cost-effectiveness accounting as well as the application of nonquantitative formal criteria for evaluating outcomes. Described in this limited way, the commitment to excellence that is included in the normative concept of managerial professionalism may be called the commitment to excellence in technique or the commitment to formal excellence. Conspicuously absent from this conception of excellence is any direct reference to the good of those clients, customers, or constituents who are to be affected by the exercise of these techniques of practical rationality.

I also suggested, however, that at least in those organizations that are understood to serve customers or clients (or in the case of a governmental bureaucracy, a constituency) the commitment to excellence goes beyond the commitment to technique. It also includes a commitment to providing the best possible product or service, within the constraints of an acceptable bottom line. To distinguish it from the mere commitment to formal excellence, let us call this the commitment to the client, customer, or constituent, or, more briefly, the service commitment. In the discourse of business, the phrase "loyalty to the customer" is often used to refer to this commitment to excellence.

The distinction between the commitment to formal excellence and the commitment to service excellence is crucial for the debate over the ethical soundness of managed care. Clearly, if managerial professionalism in the managed care context includes only the commitment to formal excellence, then the normative structure of managed care organizations is not even in principle able to accommodate what we value most in the traditional medical professional ethos: the commitment to providing high-quality care. Conversely, if the normative concept of managerial professional ethics, as it is applied to managed care, goes beyond the commitment to formal excellence to provide a central place for the commitment to service, then, at least in principle, managerial professionalism can accommodate the ideal of quality care.

There are two ways to understand the relationship between the commitment to formal excellence and the commitment to service excellence as they pertain to the normative concept of managerial professionalism. According to the first, the commitment to formal excellence is an essential element of the normative concept of managerial professionalism, but the service commitment is not, even in those cases where the organization in which the professional manager works is one that serves identifiable clients or customers, as is the case with a managed care organization. In this first view, the commitment to service excellence is optional; it is not, strictly speaking, an ethical obligation (unless the individual manager, or her organization's policy, explicitly undertakes it as such). We will call this the narrow conception of the commitment to excellence in managerial professionalism.

According to a broader conception of the commitment to excellence, managerial professionals in any bureaucratic organization that serves customers or clients have an obligation to strive not only for formal excellence but for service excellence as well. In the broader conception, managers in managed care organizations that did not honor the commitment to quality care but who simply strove for formal excellence in the pursuit of corporate profits or personal advancement would be ethically criticizable. Moreover, they would be ethically criticizable according to the standards of conduct that are internal to their identity as managerial professionals.

I am inclined to say that the normative concept of a professional manager includes the commitment not only to formal excellence but also to service excellence, at least when that concept is applied to managers working in organizations that have identifiable clients or customers. However, I would not wish to put too much weight on this analytic claim. Instead, perhaps a better way to put the central point would be this: there is a familiar and coherent normative conception of managerial professionalism that includes a commitment not only to formal excellence but to service excellence as well; if this conception is applied to the role of professional manager in managed care organizations, then managed care organizations, as a kind of bureaucratic organization, do have an ethical structure that provides a central place for the commitment to quality care. Moreover, this commitment to quality care is an intrinsic value for managers in such organizations, one whose validity does not depend solely on the instrumental value of providing quality care as a means toward maximizing profits. If this conclusion is correct, then we have a positive answer to our primary question: Is the ethics of managed care compatible with the most basic tenet of medical ethics? It is compatible, so far as managerial professionals and physicians working within managed care share a common obligation to provide the best care possible within the constraints of an acceptable bottom line.

Notice that this way of formulating what is common to the ethical obligations of physicians and managers in managed care is framed at a very general level of abstraction. All I have said is that at the most basic level the ethical task of physicians and managers is the same: to help ensure that patients get the best care possible, compatible with the financial flourishing of the organization and hence with honoring financial obligations to employees and shareholders. This common general obligation is compatible with a division of roles within managed care, which assigns different obligations of a more concrete sort to managers and physicians respectively. It may turn out, for example, that the best way to meet the shared obligation to provide quality care is for physicians to be somewhat insulated from having to make bedside rationing decisions of certain sorts or to be free of certain types of direct and powerful financial incentives to limit utilization. Whether or not this is so will depend upon what the facts are, and the facts will vary depending upon other features of particular organizations and patient populations. Here I am concerned only with articulating the general structure of ethical obligations in managed care and to compare them to familiar ideals of physician conduct.

What Is an "Acceptable Bottom Line"?

So far, the shared obligation of physicians and managers in managed care has been characterized rather vaguely as providing the best care compatible with an acceptable bottom line. The main conclusion of the analysis thus far has been that at this general level of description the chief ethical tasks of managers and physicians are not only compatible but identical. The implication is that the admittedly painful ethical predicament in which physicians find themselves in managed care is far from novel—it is in fact the recurrent ethical predicament of ethical people in business.

Now it is necessary to enrich and complicate our picture of the ethics of managed care by exploring in more detail the scope and limits of the obligation to provide quality care. The problem is to understand whether, or in what sense, the obligation to provide the best care possible and the obligation to help achieve an acceptable bottom line can be balanced.

Our earlier taxonomy of the obligations of persons in bureaucratic organizations provides a useful starting point. There we noted that whatever general obligations individuals have are not undercut simply because they take on new obligations by assuming organizational roles. Similarly, the fact that one has (general) obligations not to harm innocent persons and not to lie is not changed by having formed a particular professional identity, by committing oneself to the ideals of a particular organization's mission statement or informal corporate culture, or by the fact that one comes to have various contractual obligations in one's work as part of an organization. So whatever commitment a manager in a managed care organization has to serving the financial interests of the organization's employees and shareholders cannot be understood as negating either his general ethical obligations or his special contractual obligations. Instead, quite apart from the commitment to serving patients' interests that is part of the commitment to excellence, a manager's pursuit of a favorable bottom line is already significantly limited by general ethical obligations and by special contractual obligations incurred in the process of performing one's organizational role.

We are now in a position to state our question more precisely. Suppose that a manager or a team of managers is confronted with a choice among organizational policies or a choice among options for applying an existing policy to a particular situation or a choice among actions that will affect a patient's welfare where existing policies give no clear guidance. Suppose also that each option is compatible with fulfilling all relevant general obligations and is consistent with whatever special contractual obligations have been incurred with all legal requirements, including obligations of informed consent (understood broadly as recognition of the competent patient's right to accept or refuse treatment). Suppose also, however, that one option will maximize profitability while providing less than what would be optimal from the standpoint of the patient's interests, whereas the other option will be optimal from the standpoint of the patient's interests but suboptimal from the standpoint of profitability. What is the manager (or team of managers) obligated to do?

The answer will depend upon two factors. First, what is at stake? If a particular option would fall short of being optimal from the standpoint of the patient's interests without imposing a serious risk on him, but the alternative would spell financial disaster for the organization, then maximizing profitability may be acceptable and even obligatory, so long as the care the patient gets falls within the range of care that satisfies the standard of good medical practice—if there is a standard of good medical practice that is relevant.

The standard of good medical practice, of course, is not determined by the policies and practices of the organization in question anymore than it was determined by the behavior of any particular physician in the unmanaged fee-for-service setting. Instead, what is good medical practice must be inferred from the preponderant behavior of competent physicians in the light of the best widely accepted clinical and scientific literature. Now the character of the dominant form of health care delivery and reimbursement to some extent shapes what comes to be regarded as good medical practice. And in this sense, the standard of good medical practice does not provide a wholly independent ethical safeguard, even in principle, on the managers' commitments to pursuing profits. However, at least at present, there are several factors that shape the standard of good medical practice that are relatively independent of what might otherwise come to be standard practice in managed care. Most importantly, there are the impact (perceived or real) of malpractice litigation and the official endorsements of medical specialty organizations through consensus conferences and other scientifically informed efforts to determine what treatments are most efficacious. Thus, how significant a limitation of the commitment to providing care that meets a minimal standard of good medical practice turns out to be on the pursuit of profit-maximization will depend in part upon the extent to which the medical profession and the courts preserve an effective independent voice concerning what counts as quality care.

The second factor relevant to determining what the manager's obligations are, all things considered, is the legitimate expectations of the patient or patients who will be affected by the choice. In some cases, what the patient legitimately expects may not be limited to what is explicit in the formal terms of his or her policy. Organizational practices and the actions of particular individuals in organizations can give rise to such expectations. Although it cannot be assumed that they always represent obligations in a strict sense, nor that they override the manager's obligations to her fellow employees or stockholders, legitimate expectations must be added to the moral scales. What the ethically sound choice will be will depend not only upon these two factors, but also often upon the concrete particulars of the case. Hence no general answer to the question of how to reconcile the commitment to patient welfare and financial pressures is possible. The main point, however, is that a proper understanding of the ethics of bureaucratic organizations provides significant restrictions on the pursuit of profit and avoids the simplistic conclusion that if health care is conducted as a business then the only constraints on the pursuit of profit are fear of legal liability and a poor corporate image.

For present purposes this simplified sketch of the ethics of bureaucratic organizations and of the special ethical structure of managed care organizations must suffice. If the sketch is even roughly accurate, then there is a strong prima facie case for concluding that there is no incompatibility in principle between managed care and an intrinsic commitment on the part of those working in managed care (including physicians) to provide high-quality care. However, in order to say with more confidence that the ethics of medical professionals as we have known it can be accommodated within the organizational structure of managed care, we must first determine more precisely what it is, if anything, about the physician-patient relationship that is supposed to be both distinctive of it and incompatible with the demands that managed care organizations place on physicians.

Physician "Dedication" and the Pursuit of Financial Gain

What I shall call the traditional view of the patient-physician relationship depicts the physician as "dedicated first and foremost to serving the needs of their patients," to use the language of the American Medical Association Judicial Council's report on the ethical issues in managed care. As the report also claims, "The foundation of the patient-physician relationship is the trust that physicians will put the patient's interests first." Defenders of the traditional view typically emphasize the beneficial effects of patient trust in physicians. Trust is said to enable the patient to disclose sensitive information about herself that the physician needs to know to allay the patient's anxieties and even to enhance the efficacy of the therapies the physician offers. (Nowhere, to my knowledge, do those who cite the beneficial effects of patient trust in support of the traditional view ask what the negative effects of this trust are, much less whether the positive effects outweigh the negative ones. One negative effect worth considering is that a patient who trusts a physician when he or she shouldn't may die as a result.)

Given this understanding of the relationship, it is an easy step to frame the chief ethical issue of managed care as follows: Will the incentives to which physicians are subjected in managed care undermine the physician's dedication to putting the patient's interests first and hence undermine patient trust, with the result that the beneficial effects of patient trust will be lost?

In this context, "the physician's dedication to putting the patient's interests first" is taken to refer to a motivational fact about physicians (or most physicians, at any rate). The putative fact is that they characteristically subordinate their own interests (and the interests of third parties) to those of their patients when these interests are in conflict. In simplest terms, the claim is that the physician's (most physicians') motivation to do what is best for the patient dominates all other motivations, including the physician's pursuit of her own financial well-being or other interests.

Notice that we must understand the claim as a claim about the actual efficacy of the physician's commitment to the patient's interests (rather than as a claim about how physicians ought to act), unless we are to interpret the statement that it is essential to preserve patient trust in an utterly cynical fashion. For only if (at least for the most part) the physician's commitment to the patient's interest is dominant in fact (not just in the ideals of traditional medical ethics) will the patient's trust in that commitment be warranted. Otherwise, whatever efficacy patient trust may have is founded on an illusion.

Now I wish to ask a question that some may at first tend to dismiss as absurd or at least disrespectful of the medical profession: What reason is there to believe that most physicians do have an actually dominant commitment to the patient's best interest? Clearly, neither the fact that they are enjoined to have such a commitment by traditional medical ethics nor the fact that they are said to have it counts as sufficient evidence, or indeed as any evidence at all, that they in fact do. To my knowledge, there are no scientific data to support this very strong empirical generalization about the motivational makeup of physicians as a class.

Remember what is at issue here is a claim about the strength of a particular motive or commitment. Hence the best evidence that the motivation to act in the patient's best interest is actually dominant—is in fact sufficiently strong that it typically determines the individual's behavior in spite of contrary motives or commitments—would be a preponderance of actual instances in which contrary motives were present, but the physician acted in the patient's best interests nonetheless. If contrary motivations were not present or if circumstances ensured that even if present such contrary motivations were relatively weak, then the mere fact that the physician in the past acted in the patient's best interest would not be good evidence that he had a dominant disposition to act so nor, therefore, for a prediction that he would do so in the future.

Unfortunately for those who assume that physicians put the patient's interest first, the very conditions of practice under which physicians have operated, from the dominance of the unmanaged, third-party fee-for-service system until very recently, have made it difficult to find evidence to support the empirical generalization that physicians put the patient's interests first. For the great achievement of the traditional third-party fee-for-service system was that it achieved a high degree of congruence between the patient's best (medical) interest on the one hand and the physician's interest in financial gain (and professional autonomy) on the other. (The congruence was not perfect, of course, because the system gave incentives for overutilization, which sometimes resulted in unnecessary pain and discomfort or iatrogenic injuries and diseases.) But, generally speaking, the physician's pursuit of her own financial gain and her dedication to the patient's best (medical) interest spoke as with one voice in the unmanaged, third-party fee-for-service system.

To put the same point differently, the old system economized on physician altruism. The incentives of the unmanaged, third-party fee-for-service system financially rewarded the physician for doing what he or she believed was in the patient's best (medical) interest.

Under these conditions, little dedication to the patient's interests and little if any financial sacrifice on the part of the physician were required. But for this very reason, the behavior of physicians under the old system can provide scant evidence that physicians as a group, and on average, have an actually dominant motivation to act in their patients' best interests. In a system that economizes on altruism, evidence of exceptionally altruistic motivation will be lacking.

To summarize, in order to support the claim that physicians are dedicated to putting the patient's interest first, it is not sufficient to show that they have generally acted in the patient's best interest if they have done so in a system that achieves a high degree of congruence between their own financial interests and their patients' interests. As an empirical generalization about the relative strength (or comparative efficacy) of the commitment to patient welfare, the traditional view's declaration of physician dedication was simply not tested by the old system. Ironically, it is only with the advent of managed care, in which the congruence between the physician's financial interests and the patient's best interest can be broken, that we are in a position to test the empirical generalization about physician motivation or commitment upon which the traditional view rests and that for many has framed the debate about the ethics of managed care.

Here a disclaimer is necessary. My contention is not that there is no evidence available of physician altruism. There are no doubt instances of physician altruism, just as there are instances of plumber and auto mechanic altruism. My point, rather, is that the nature of the system of reimbursement that has existed until recently is such that we cannot take the fact that physicians generally act in the patient's (medical) interests as sound evidence that they put the patient's interest first if this means that they have a dominant motivation to serve the patient's interest. Nor does the fact (assuming it is a fact) that physicians in the old system generally acted in the best (medical) interests of their patients show that physicians as a group are any more dedicated to service than other professionals, or other vendors of goods or services for that matter.

Like lawyers, plumbers, and auto mechanics, physicians faced certain conflicts of interests, even in the old system. Regardless of the fact that the physician was being reimbursed for providing her services, she frequently faced choices about the intensity or timing of services, where one option maximized the patient's interest, but another was more convenient for the physician or enabled the physician to better honor her commitments to other patients or to her family. But to say that when faced with such choices physicians sometimes put the patient's interest first is a far cry from showing that they typically do or that they do so more often than others, such as lawyers, plumbers, or auto mechanics. To my knowledge there are no data to show that physicians as a group are any more altruistic in these matters than other folk.

This is not a criticism. It is only a reminder that the statement that physicians "put the patient's interest first" is only literally true if it is understood as a normative or aspirational statement about how physicians ideally ought to act rather than as a description of how they (or most of them, most of the time) do act. As a description of how physicians do act—and it is only thus that it can serve as a rational basis for patient trust—the statement that physicians are dedicated to their patients or that they put their patients' interests first is at best unsubstantiated and at worst false if it means that whenever other interests conflict with the patient's best interest, the physician pursues only the latter.

Instead, it seems better to understand the statement that physicians put their patients' interests first as aspirational—as an imperative, an exhortation to physicians as to what their priorities ought to be. But notice that it would be unreasonable, as well as unrealistic, to expect physicians literally to put their patients' interests first all the time, no matter how weighty the conflicting obligations to family or friends are. Indeed, it would not even be reasonable (whether it would be realistic or not) to expect physicians always to subordinate their own (purely self-regarding) interests.

Similarly, when we say that parents ought to put their children's interest first, we do not literally mean it. We do not mean that in every instance the parent ought to sacrifice her own interests, no matter how important, to those of her child. After all, parents have lives to lead too. At most what is meant is that the parent ought to accord an exceptional priority to the child's more important interests and that a greater degree of selflessness is required of parents in their behavior toward their children than is mandatory in human interactions generally, including interactions with those to whom we have no such intimate connection. So being a good parent does not mean always acting in the child's best interest, that is, literally optimizing the child's welfare.

Likewise, it would be as inappropriate to require of physicians that they literally put their patients' interest first in every instance (in the sense of doing only that which optimizes the patient's welfare) as it would be erroneous to believe that physicians actually do always put their patients' interests first. But if this is the case, then it will not do to say that although physicians have an absolute commitment to the patient's interest, the ethics of a managed care organization falls short of this because it only exhorts employees to provide the best care compatible with an acceptable bottom line. Neither the physician's obligation to serve his patient's interest nor the manager's obligation to provide quality service is absolute. Both make room for balancing the commitment to the patient, within limits, against other interests and obligations.

Why Deflating the Myth of Physician "Dedication" Makes a Difference

I have taken some pains to show that we ought not take at face value the traditional claim that physicians put their patients' interest first if by this is meant that physicians do in fact always subordinate other interests, including their own, to the patient's best interest. I have also argued that we have no sound evidence for concluding that physicians are, relatively speaking, more dedicated toward those whom they serve than other professionals. But if this is correct, then it follows that one common way of framing the ethical issues in managed care ought to be rejected out of hand. We should not assume that the problem is how to preserve the physician's dedication to the patient in the face of the contrary incentives of managed care. To state the issue in this way is to assume what we are not entitled to assume, either that until now physicians have in fact had a dominant motivation to act in the patient's best interests or that being an ethical physician requires that one always optimize patient welfare.

Because we lack sufficient evidence for the first factual claim, we should not bank on strategies for coping with the conflicts of interest that rely on the assumption that there is a strong reservoir of physician altruism whose purity and bounty need only be maintained. Because the ethical obligations of physicians to their patients (like those of parents toward their children) do not require that they always act in the best interest of their patients, we should not assume that a reasonable concern about the financial bottom line is incompatible with being an ethical physician. The challenge, rather, is to achieve as close congruence as possible between an organization that is functioning well in the marketplace and high-quality patient care. In evaluating various strategies for doing this we cannot assume that the main criterion of evaluation is how well such strategies preserve physician altruism, because we have no basis for attributing exceptional altruism to physicians in the first place. Nor should we look for strategies that will allow physicians to act only in the patient's best interests, because medical ethics does not require that they do so.

Status Trust versus Merit Trust

It was noted earlier that, in the traditional conception of the patient-physician relationship, the patient's trust in the physician is assumed (without data or argument) to be of significant net benefit—that its benefits outweigh its risks. We now must focus more closely on exactly what sort of trust this is supposed to be and upon what precisely it is supposed to be based. Only by doing so can we hope to ascertain whether the shift to managed care will undermine trust and, if so, whether that will be a bad thing.

I have already argued that the empirical generalization that (most) physicians have a dominant motivation to further their patients' interests is at present unsubstantiated. So if the basis of patient trust is this empirical generalization, then this trust is misplaced. This is not to say, of course, that it is irrational for any particular patient to trust his or her physician. The question is, rather, what is the basis of the trust?

Two quite distinct types of trust should be distinguished: status trust and merit trust. The kind of trust celebrated by the traditional view of the patient-physician relationship is status trust. Status trust exists when the mere perception that an individual has a certain status (or role) results in others' placing some significant degree of trust in that individual (or, put negatively, in others' suspending critical attitudes and self-protective strategies that they would ordinarily exhibit in their interpersonal activities). To trust a doctor because he or she is a doctor, independent of any evidence concerning the actual competence or integrity of this particular doctor, is to accord that individual status trust.

In many societies, and in ours until recently, status trust has been accorded to teachers, military officers, physicians or healers, priests, and even government officials. Probably for most of this century, though not necessarily before that, the medical profession in this country has enjoyed considerable status trust. However, one can accord status trust by degrees. To place some trust in an individual simply because he or she is a doctor is not necessarily to trust without limit.

Merit trust, in contrast, is trust based on beliefs about the actual performance and character of the individual, not just on his or her status as a member in a professional or occupational group. Merit trust may be direct or derivative. A businessperson who has gained the trust of others by repeatedly acting honestly and responsibly toward them is a recipient of direct merit trust. A person who is trusted because he is a member of an organization that has merited one's trust is a recipient of derivative trust.

This distinction between status trust and merit trust is important because it enables us to avoid a false dilemma that constrains and distorts much of the debate over the ethics of managed care. The false dilemma is that we must choose between a system in which health care is conducted as a business and one in which patients trust their physicians. The erroneous assumption underlying the alleged dilemma is that trust is unique to the patient-physician relationship and that it does not play a significant role in business. Although it may be true that one particular kind of trust—status trust—has played a distinctive role in health care until now, it is also true that another kind of trust—merit trust—has always played a crucial role in business.

There are two reasons not to mourn the erosion of patient trust, if what is meant by this is status trust. First, excessive or misplaced status trust is a very dangerous and costly thing, and it is in the nature of status trust that some who are accorded it will not deserve it. Most of us now recognize that it is imprudent if not irresponsible to place a great deal of trust in an individual simply because he or she is a physician. The growing popularity of second opinions, not just among insurers eager to reduce unnecessary surgery but also among consumers, is one instance of the increasing recognition that status trust toward physicians can be imprudent. Second, it is not a matter of status trust or no trust at all. There is much to be said for not trusting physicians (or plumbers or lawyers) unless they merit it, either through our direct acquaintance with their proficiency and reliability or on the basis of the reputation of the organization for which they work.

Changing to a system in which status trust is largely replaced by merit trust is not changing to a system in which there is no trust between patient and physician. Moreover, there is certainly room for merit trust of physicians in managed care, merit trust of both the direct and the derivative sort. And there is no reason to think that whatever benefits status trust provides cannot be provided by merit trust.

This is not to say that it will be an easy thing for managed care organizations to achieve merit trust. They will not be able to achieve, or at least to sustain, it unless they can convince consumers that they are doing a good job of achieving a congruence between providing the best care and securing an acceptable bottom line. But as I noted earlier, this problem is not unique to managed care; it is the central challenge for businesses generally.

Is the Ethics of Business Organizations Compatible with the Ethical Practice of Medicine?

Physicians can act ethically while still functioning well as members of managed care organizations if these organizations reward and encourage ethical behavior and penalize and discourage unethical behavior. I have argued that one would only assume that managed care organizations as such are incapable of doing this if one had a mistaken view of the nature of business and of the ethics of organizations. Once we reject clumsy dichotomies that present physicians as exceptional altruists and business people as relentless pursuers of profit, constrained only by fear of legal liability and a poor corporate image, we can see that the ethics of business organizations makes room for most if not all that we value in the physician-patient relationship. Most importantly, the ethics of business organizations, as it is commonly understood, provides a central place for a commitment to excellence in the provision of health care, where this includes the commitment to patient welfare.

This is not to say, however, that the task of creating and sustaining an ethical health care business is anything less than enormously difficult and complex. Nor is it to say that business people always act ethically or to deny that in bureaucratic organizations operating in extremely competitive environments (whether their legal status is for-profit or nonprofit) there are exceptionally strong incentives to act unethically. It is to say, however, that there is a place, an honored place, for the physician—and others—within the managed care organization to act as the patient's advocate, just as there is room for a service manager to act as her customer's advocate or a corporate lawyer to act as her client's advocate. Only if one (falsely) assumed that the only sort of attainable (or beneficial) trust is status trust or that only medical professionals have an intrinsic, noninstrumental commitment to excellence would one conclude that there is a fundamental incompatibility between managed care and patient trust based on a reasonable, though not unlimited, commitment to the patient's interest.

Let me emphasize that the purpose of this article has not been to solve the problems of conflict of interest that arise in managed care. Instead, my goal has been to help clear the way for such solutions by disposing of a mistaken and constraining assumption about the incompatibility of what is most valuable in medical ethics and the operation of an ethical managed care enterprise. My main point is that, given a sufficiently rich conception of the ethics of organizations, including business organizations, there is no fundamental incompatibility.

Having said this, I would conclude by pointing out that there are some ethical challenges for which they may be singularly unprepared that physicians will increasingly face as managed care becomes the dominant form of health care delivery. Recall that I assumed at the outset that the transition to managed care is best characterized as a shift from a system of health care delivery in which physicians largely operated free of organizational constraints and in which medical professionalism dominated to one in which physicians were significantly constrained by organizational demands and in which managerial professionalism held sway. If this is so then one would expect that physicians as a group are relatively inexperienced in coping with some of the most common ethical problems that arise in bureaucratic organizations—in particular what I referred to earlier as the ethics of exit, voice, and loyalty (conscientious refusal and resignation, whistle-blowing, and the like). If this is so, then traditional medical ethics may be of very limited use in coping with some of the most challenging ethical problems arising from the new realities of medical practice.

Moreover, if, as I have argued, business has its own ethical principles and traditions, then physicians who dismiss "mere businesspeople" as ethical primitives may in fact be cutting themselves off from a rich source of practical knowledge for coping with their new predicament.

CHAPTER 3

Whether to Discontinue Nonfutile Use of a Scarce Resource

Frances M. Kamm

IN THIS ESSAY I consider some of the ethical problems presented by the desire to discontinue the nonfutile use of scarce resources. It is said that doctors should not do "rationing at the bedside" with patients. Rather, rationing should result from a systemwide macro-policy that ties their hands. However, I shall argue there may be an in-between case: When individuals are involved in trials for use of drugs, treatment to them might be discontinued because they do not do well enough, if and only if treating those who do better makes it possible to treat more candidates who are equally worthy. The drug clozapine, uniquely useful for treating schizophrenia, is taken as an example of such a resource made scarce because of its costliness.[1]

In the first section of the essay I consider relevant available medical data, and I review current treatment policy involving the drug. In subsequent sections I isolate three major issues that arise in the morality of discontinuing aid: regression, doctors' commitments to patients, and the temporal gap between denying aid to one person and providing better aid to someone else; I also deal with whether differential outcome should affect who gets helped. To examine this topic, I present in outline some general principles for the distribution of scarce resources[2] and then begin to make clear what these principles might imply for the case of differential outcomes with clozapine. The concluding sections consider the role of differential numbers of people who might be helped and the significance of urgency relative to outcome. I attempt to provide a morally justified principle that tells us how to relate the *outcome* we expect in treating patients to the *urgency* of patients' conditions and the *number* of potential recipients of treatment. The final section of the essay considers the fate of those individuals who are only moderately ill and suggests a possible change in policy that might be of benefit in achieving just distribution to them.

Background

Suppose that clozapine is currently the most effective treatment for schizophrenia, helping people who would not otherwise be helped, helping them more

55

than alternative treatments do, and causing fewer side effects. However, suppose it is more expensive than other treatments, at least in the short run. Whether it is more expensive in the long run than other treatments depends upon the outcomes it provides.

In some people, clozapine treatment essentially results in a return to normality. These people can leave hospitals so hospital beds can be eliminated. Such patients must continue to take medication costing about $5,500 per year. But they can become self-supporting, returning to work and family. This implies they themselves could fund their medication (via private insurance). In this population, clozapine is overall less expensive than other treatments.

Other people show only moderate improvement, both in the sense that the difference between their condition with clozapine and without it is not great and in the sense that they do not return to normality. These individuals must continue the drug in order to get benefits that only clozapine can provide to them, but they cannot live independently. They may move to outpatient facilities supported by both state and federal funds, or they may have to remain in state-run hospitals. In this population, clozapine use is overall more expensive than other treatments.

In a third group, clozapine produces no differential benefits, and its use typically is not indicated. However, the possibility that it produces fewer side effects, even if it is no more effective than other treatments, raises the question of whether its use is nonetheless indicated.

Suppose that there is no way to tell before treatment into which of these three groups a person will fall. For example, there is an equal distribution of big successes (normality) in severe and nonsevere patients. However, once someone is on treatment, one can tell within six months whether that person will respond, and to what degree.

Assume that when clozapine must be provided at public expense it is a scarce resource owing to its costliness. A significant ethical problem that arises is whether to continue treating those who cannot pay for their own treatment and who make only moderate gains that do not lift them to normality. This is one of the most expensive groups to treat, and discontinuing their treatment would allow us to help more people become normal. In other words, should the maintenance of someone on the scarce resource depend on the outcome it produces?

At present, it is said,[3] the publicly funded treatment policy being followed is essentially twofold: (1) Keep on treating all those who achieve normality on the drug (indeed, this is taken for granted). (2) Give medication in accordance with the severity of the illness and *keep on* treating even those who improve only to a subnormal level. This means that others who are not so severely ill but who might achieve normality are not treated. For prongs (1) and (2) of this policy to be consistent, it must be assumed that most of the normals who are continued on treatment would otherwise be severely ill, even if not all the severely ill who are treated attain normality.

Issues Specific to Discontinuing Treatment

The decision to stop treating those who are achieving a moderate level of well-being—the rejection of prong (2)—in order to try to increase the number who can achieve normality raises several ethical questions. The first asks: Is there a moral difference between (a) not beginning treatment that would help someone achieve only a moderate level of well-being in order to help others more, and (b) terminating such treatment once it has begun in order to help others more? All the issues (for example, concerning action and omission) that are familiar from the discussion of discontinuing life-sustaining treatment might be thought to arise here. It might be said, however, that *not* giving yet another dose of a drug is not the same as terminating (by action) a life-support system. At most, it is like a case involving a life-support machine that needs to be reset every day. Then the issue is also whether it is permissible to omit resetting it.

Whatever the philosophically best way to treat the termination-versus-not-beginning-treatment issue may be, psychological studies might support the view that if people form *expectations* about future treatment on the basis of past treatment, this will set a baseline from which noncontinuation of treatment will be perceived as a loss.[4] For those who have not yet received treatment and have not formed expectations about getting treatment, not being treated may be perceived as a no-gain situation. Losses tend to be ranked more negatively than "no-gains," even when they both leave the patient at the same absolute level of well-being. Would this be a reason not to terminate drug use, even when we may refuse to begin it? It is possible that one could prevent the development of expectations concerning further treatment by explicitly warning people that beginning treatment does not guarantee that treatment will continue. Then the expectation of treatment would not be a reason to continue, for there would be no expectation. Furthermore, ceasing treatment should then be seen as a no-gain rather than a loss. Deliberately characterizing the first six months of use of the drug as a *trial* may succeed in stemming expectations.

However, there might be other determinative reasons against stopping treatment. For example, if we are clear about what terminating treatment with clozapine leads to in a patient we may see another ground for objecting to it. Theoretically, there are two possibilities for the trial: (a) treatment must be continued for up to six months in order for us to know (by some sign) whether someone will become normal but there is no change in the patient's condition during that time period; (b) treatment must be continued for up to six months in order for us to know whether someone will become normal and there is an improvement in the patient's condition during that time period. I believe it is (b) rather than (a) that raises a moral problem for terminating treatment. In (b), terminating treatment does not merely stop a patient from achieving further progress (as it may in [a]); it allows the patient to regress, to fall back down to the level from which he or she was already lifted. It is not stopping treatment per se, even when we know this will prevent some future improvement that seems morally significant relative to not starting treatment. What seems morally significant is *stopping an improvement in the patient's condition that has already occurred by stopping what was being done to achieve it.* The latter condition is important. For suppose a regress would occur unless we increase the dosage already given. I do not believe that refusing to prevent the regress in order to help others instead would raise the same concern. Hence, it is not even the regress per se but its occurrence as a result of not continuing to do what was already being done that may be problematic. (Call this regression*.)

This concern with regression* assumes that improvement to a point below normality is still better than being in a much worse condition. Some may challenge this assumption. They may point out that some individuals who are severely mentally ill live in a world of pleasant delusions. When patients recover partially, they become aware of their problems and for the first time experience misery. Several points can be made in response to this challenge. First, if severely ill schizophrenics are already very miserable, the challenge does not apply to them. Second, the challenge depends on a completely experiential conception of the good life: What you do not experience as bad is not bad for you and there are no nonexperiential goods that compensate for experiential harms. If this were a correct conception of the good life, it would imply that a good life could be had by taking drugs that give one pleasant experiences and the illusion of living a productive life. It also denies that pain experienced in coming into contact with reality can be compensated by the mere fact that one is in contact with reality. There is much to be said against the experiential conception of the good life.

Let us now consider a doctor's point of view on stopping treatment that involves regression*. A doctor who omits to continue the same treatment may view herself as fully responsible for the decline in the patient and think that "producing" this decline is worse than not aiding the patient to start with. Yet a philosopher might reasonably argue that it is as permissible (or impermissible) not to continue aid that one had been providing as it is not to start aid even if the patient declines, as long as she declines to a state that is no worse than she would have been in if aid had not begun, assuming there is no independent commitment (e.g., a promise) to continue aid once started. But is one worse off if one improves for a few months and then declines than if one had never improved at all? I do not believe so, for if all we could ever do for any patient was improve him for a few months before an inevitable decline, doing so would be better for him than not.

Admittedly, a doctor has a duty to aid (unlike an ordinary bystander), but even with this duty, a doctor may refuse to start helping one patient in order to help a greater number of other patients. Why then may she not stop the aid once started, in order to help others more, if the patient will be no worse off overall and being in the trial gave him a chance for continued treatment? Must the fact that the patient gets worse again through failure to continue what has already been done be definitive? I suggest not.

It is also inappropriate to apply the Hippocratic doctor's concern with not doing harm above all to the case of the patient's decline. First, the doctor would be refusing to continue aiding, and this is not, strictly, harming. Furthermore, looking only at what happens if we do not continue to aid relative to the patient's improved condition considers too narrow a time slice; it fails to consider the overall period from before the doctor intervened: the doctor produced the improvement and would not have been duty-bound to do so if he could alternatively have helped more people. Not helping someone retain an improvement and instead helping others may be aesthetically less pleasing than not helping to start with—declines to a level may be less pleasing than maintenance of a status quo at that same level—but it is not clear that it is morally different.

This brings us to another objection to terminating treating based on the idea that a doctor might simply become committed to a specific patient once treatment starts. I do not believe that this gives rise to an obligation to continue aid in all cases. Commitments may be overridden, for example, by the attempt to help greater numbers of people, especially if these are also one's patients. In addition, commitments could be undertaken by doctors in an explicitly conditional form, for example: "You will be provided with a drug, on condition no one else needs it more." It may be part of the *responsibility of patients* (correlative to their rights) to accept that their useful treatment may be stopped for morally legitimate reasons. Most importantly, the idea of a commitment to a patient suggests that a doctor would be wrong to stop treatment that had not yet had *any* effect on the patient when the doctor knows that continuing treatment will lead to some subnormal improvement in the future. But I do not believe the doctor would be wrong to drop treatment for such a patient in order to offer it to others who can reach normality. All this suggests that it is regression* that raises the moral problem, not simple failure of commitment or simply termination of treatment.

It is true, however, that playing down a doctor's commitment to individual patients makes the establishment of special bonds (comparable to the ones we form with friends or family members) impossible. Such special bonds are thought legitimately to impede meeting even the more pressing needs of other people. Should we exchange the possibility of such bonds between doctor and patient for fairer treatment? The suggestion is that we could morally afford to do so by having trials that can be ended.

Nevertheless, there are particular facts of the clozapine case that further complicate the decision not to continue aid to someone in order to help others more. Terminating aid so as to *definitely help* others more is different from terminating aid to *go searching* for others who will do better. In the latter case, we cannot be sure that we will be helping the next person more than we are helping the person already being treated and it will take up to six months to find out. The person on whom we try our next drug may do no better, and possibly worse, than the person we dropped. If he does worse, this means that we could have been doing more good by having continued treatment for the first patient. What if he and subsequent trial subjects do only as well as the person dropped? It might be argued that this is still a better outcome, for there is a fairer distribution of temporary moderate improvements. For example, instead of n months of moderate improvement going to one person, m patients get n/m months of moderate improvement. If we had to distribute the good of moderate improvement to begin with, we might well divide it over several people rather than concentrate its duration in one person, as long as what we distribute is still a significant good. (Notice that this is not the same as saying that we would deny normality to someone by dividing a normality-producing dose so as to produce only moderate well-being in many.) Regression*, admittedly, might be the dominate countervailing consideration to such a fairer distribution of moderate improvement.

Still, there is at least a chance that the drug will prove *very* successful in the next person, and this is no longer true of the person we would drop. The probability of finding people who do much better is an empirical question, and we may be reluctant to stop helping one person unless there is a sufficiently high probability of helping others much more in the *near future*.

This last point makes salient the time gap that can exist between stopping aid to one person and finding another person whom we can help reach normality. At worst, it is possible that by the time we find someone who does better and help him, we may no longer be helping someone who was suffering at the same time as the person we originally dropped. If this is so, we will have put off helping someone who is suffering *now* with the consequence that we help others more who will suffer *in the future*. This raises the question of whether we should adopt an attitude of *temporal neutrality*, not distinguishing between those who need help now and those who will come with need later. (I shall return to a related issue below.)

Severity, Outcome, and a General Theory of Distribution

Here is another ethical question raised by the decision not to continue treatment of those who are achieving moderate well-being in order to increase the number of individuals who can achieve normality: Should the attempt to achieve normality for some lead us to deprive others of their chance for moderate improvement, even if these others are more severely ill than those who would be substituted for them in drug trials? This question arises independently of the possible moral problem of stopping treatment, for theoretically it could also arise in cases where we must decide whether to start aiding someone. This question has two subparts: (a) Should better outcomes dominate equal chances for help in those whose condition is equally severe? (b) Should better outcomes dominate greater severity?

In this section, I shall deal with subpart (a). It will be useful to first present some general principles for distributing scarce resources. I have elsewhere attempted to describe a distribution procedure that takes account of four factors: need (N), urgency (U), outcome (O), and waiting time (WT).[5] Factors besides these four may be relevant; however, I believe one should not start by cluttering the picture. In general, the method is to begin with one factor, holding the others constant in the background, and to see what differences variation in this factor make. Then we can vary two factors, finding out what the relation is between them—for example, which takes precedence over the other. Then we introduce a third factor to see whether its presence makes a difference to the relationship between the first two factors as well as how the third relates to each of the two others. If we follow this procedure patiently, adding additional factors in an orderly way, we have some hope of making progress.

Let me first describe three of the four factors N, U, and O. A patient's *urgency* (U), as I use the term, is a measure of how bad his future prospects are if he is not treated; it is a function of how bad this future will be and the likelihood it will come about. (This is not the ordinary notion of urgency, which also focuses on how soon treatment is needed. Someone could face very bad prospects but not need treatment to avoid such prospects as soon as someone else, in which case the ordinary notion says his case is not as urgent.) *Need* for treatment (N), as I use the term, connotes how badly someone's life will go overall if that person is not treated. Unlike urgency, need is not merely a forward-looking concept; it takes someone's whole life, healthwise, into consideration. Person A could be more *urgent than* B, in that A will die in a month if he is not treated now and B will die in a year if he is not treated now, and yet B could be more in need (of life-giving treatment) because he would die at age twenty whereas A would die at age eighty. This assumes that one will have had a worse life overall if one dies at twenty than if one dies at eighty (other things equal). Because need takes into account someone's past about which one can no longer do anything, it implies that how we treat someone in the future could at least compensate someone for the past, and that such compensation could be as morally important as prevention of harm in the future. (This may be a contentious assumption.)

Outcome (O) refers to the expected difference that treatment will make. In cases where life and death are at issue, I believe that the relevant measure of outcome is additional time alive independent of quality, as long as the patient would find the quality of life acceptable. This means that we should not use

QALY (quality-adjusted life years) in evaluating different possible outcomes if our focus is on helping each person as an end in itself. In cases where life and death are *not* at issue, outcome is appropriately measured in terms of (some types of) quality-of-life differences, such as relative freedom from the symptoms of schizophrenia.[6]

What are some of the things we can say about the relative weights of N, O, and U? First, let us consider distribution of a scarce, *lifesaving* resource between A and B, holding need, urgency, and outcome (as well as any other factor) constant. Fairness requires giving each an equal chance. It is important to understand that giving equal chances is *not* a symptom of the desire not to be responsible for making a choice. It is, rather, the fair way to choose when there is no morally relevant difference between potential recipients, each of whom wants to be the one to survive.

Now add a third person, C, whose need, urgency, and outcome are the same (and who can also be saved only if we save B). What I call the "balancing argument" claims that in such a case, justice demands that each person on one side should have her interests balanced against those of one person on the opposing side; those who are not balanced out in the larger group help determine that the larger group should be saved. Hence, the number of people we can save counts morally.

Now consider conflicts when the individuals are not equally urgent. Figure 3.1 represents a choice between saving A on the one hand, and, on the other hand, saving B *and* curing C's sore throat with leftover medicine. The overall outcomes will be different depending on whom we save, as more good, spread over two people, will occur if we save B and C. My claim is that we should treat the difference in outcome as morally irrelevant.

The reasoning behind this is as follows: From an impartial view, we should not favor A over B per se (given that they are assumed alike *in themselves* in all morally relevant respects). If they were alone (independent of C), we should give equal chances. From the impartial perspective, we also see that A and B each has his own partial point of view: A prefers his own survival to that of B, and vice versa. It is important to each, therefore, that he retain his equal chance to survive. The fact that we could save C from a sore throat is a matter of minor importance to him; he is not very needy or urgent and, in addition, the difference in outcome achieved by helping him is small. These three points lead to the conclusion that we should not deprive A of his fifty percent chance of survival merely to also help C. Indeed, I would conclude that C's cure should be a morally irrelevant good in choosing between these people. (This contrasts with the view that we should *aggregate* the gain to B and C and help them because we produce a benefit that is larger than the benefit to A alone.)

This form of reasoning gives equal consideration to each individual's partial point of view from an impartial point of view, so it combines subjective and

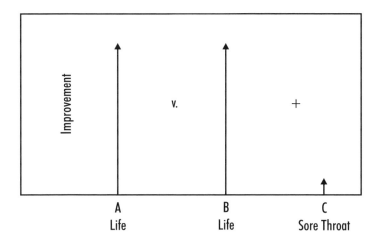

FIGURE 3.1   THE SORE THROAT CASE

objective perspectives. Hence, I call it "sobjectivity." It implies that certain goods (like the throat cure) can be morally irrelevant; I call this the "principle of irrelevant goods." Whether a good is irrelevant is context-dependent. Curing a sore throat is morally irrelevant when others' lives are at stake, but not when others' earaches are. The sore throat case shows that we must refine the claim at the base of the balancing argument that what we owe each person is to balance her interests against the equal interests of an opposing person and let the remainder help determine the outcome.

If small increases in good to a person are sometimes morally irrelevant, this can help provide one reason why someone who has a big and even irreplaceable effect on society *in aggregate* should not necessarily be favored in the distribution of a scarce lifesaving resource over someone else. If the big effect amounts to only small effects on the lives of many people, then these effects should not, I believe, be aggregated so as to help outweigh the claim of someone else to also have a fifty percent chance to have his life saved.

Aggregating small benefits to many people, *none* of whom are very needy or urgent, to outweigh the grave need of a single person can be even more problematic than aggregating saving a life and providing such small benefits in order to outweigh someone else's equal chance to live. Such a problematic procedure would be exemplified by public policies that, for example, provide marriage counseling to the great number of people who will need it rather than provide care for a far fewer number of the severely schizophrenic.

Suppose (as in figure 3.2) that if we save B rather than A, we can also save C's arm. This is the prevention of a large loss to C. I believe that when the loss to C

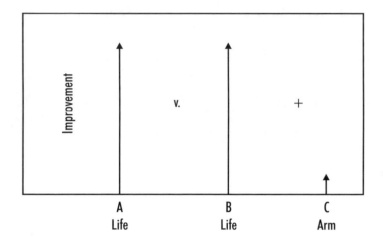

FIGURE 3.2   THE EXTRA ARM CASE

becomes so significant, it is no longer an irrelevant good, given that we can only save one life no matter what we do. This is true even though C does not stand to lose as much as A or B and so is not as needy or as urgent as each of them. Explaining why this moral shift occurs when the good to another person is large is not easy, and I shall not attempt it here. This shift would mean either that we should give the treatment outright to B and C or at least that we should give them a greater proportional chance of getting the treatment.

What if the extra good is concentrated in the person whose life would be saved? That is, suppose we could save A's or B's life, but, if we save B, we could also save him from having a sore throat, which A will suffer if she is saved. Here the need and urgency of A and B are the same, but the outcome each presents is different. My claim is that the sore throat is an irrelevant difference in a decision of life and death, and we should not deprive A of her chance to live because of it, even though no more than one person can be saved.

Suppose we could save A or B, but, if we save B, we will also prevent his arm from falling off, whereas A's arm would fall off anyway. Is the saving of an arm here a morally relevant utility that should incline us to save B rather than A? (See figure 3.3.)

I believe that B's arm is morally irrelevant. Further, I believe this is consistent with my conclusion earlier that C's arm is relevant in figure 3.2. When the improvement in quality of life would occur in the very same person for whom the primary good at stake is life itself—that is, when the good is concentrated rather than distributed—I believe the additional good we can do him should not necessarily lead us to deprive A of her chance at a life that she finds acceptable.

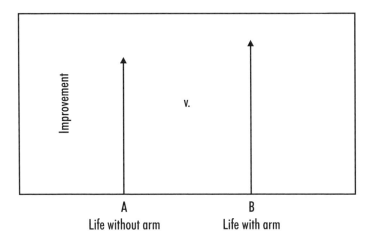

FIGURE 3.3   THE LIFE WITH AN EXTRA ARM CASE

Three principles underlie this conclusion. First, *we are more concerned with helping someone avoid being in a very bad condition than with providing the very same person whom we would help in that way with an additional improvement.* Second, *each person wants to be the one who avoids the very bad condition and come close to being normal.* (The fact that A might be willing to run a risk of death [in surgery] to be saved the loss of an arm does not imply that he would run a greater risk of death so that B can have a greater chance of being saved with both arms.)[7] Third, when an extra good is distributed over another person rather than concentrated, we positively affect a greater number of people. This is a right-making feature not present when B receives an extra good.

Finally, suppose that we have a choice between helping one person, A, who will be very badly off and much benefited by our aid, or helping a couple of people, B and C, each of whom will be as badly off as A but not benefited as much by our aid. As long as the lesser benefit is significant, it is morally more important, I think, to distribute our efforts over more people, each of whom would be as badly off as the single person, rather than to provide a bigger benefit concentrated in one person (other things being equal). One way to analyze this situation employs what I shall call "balancing argument (II)": Find the part of the potential large gain to A (part 1) that is balanced by the smaller gain to B. Now we must decide how to break the tie between them. If we care about giving priority to those who are worse off, we will care more about benefiting the next person in the group, C, rather than giving an additional benefit (part 2) to A, who, having received part 1, would already have more than C. This means that instead of breaking the tie between A-with-part-1 and B by giving A a greater benefit (part 2), we break the tie by helping two people, each to a lesser degree.

Clozapine and Differences in Outcome in a Two-Person Choice

In the case of clozapine we are considering whose quality of life to improve, not whose life to save. Again, let us assume at this point that need and urgency are great and constant among people, but that outcomes will be different. Also let us assume for the time being that the only two people affected by our choices are A and B, and they can both be improved only by clozapine. (See figure 3.4.)

Assume B will be improved *slightly* beyond A, to the point of normality. The view most clearly implied by my previous discussion is that in this case we should not deprive A of his equal chance to make what is a more critical change from a very bad condition to being close to normal, just in order to bring B first close to normal and then make the further less crucial move slightly beyond to normality. The principles that underlie this conclusion are (1) we are more concerned with helping someone avoid a very bad condition than with providing him with an additional improvement, and (2) each person wants to be the one who avoids the very bad condition.

Here is an alternative view: normal mental health (which need not mean perfect mental health) is a unique kind of good. It is closely associated with the characteristics that are commonly thought to account for the moral importance of being a person at all: rationality, self-control, capacity for responsible action, and so forth. The difference between normality and its absence is not just a mat-

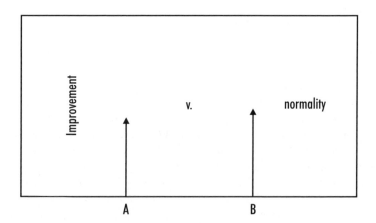

FIGURE 3.4   TWO-PERSON CHOICES: THE NORMAL PERSON CASE

ter of degree, like the difference between perfect pain relief and some degree of pain. Improvement to a moderate level of mental health is a good for the person who is ill, as is improvement to normality. But normality is also more than a good *for* the person; it helps account for the importance of being a person. Being in normal physical condition does not have a comparable role. We might, therefore, see achieving it as an especially important goal that represents more than just an additional benefit to someone who already will have achieved the most important part of what is good for him.

Call this the "mental-special view."[8] Here is a possible implication of it: Avoiding a truly horrifying mental condition could be so important that we should not deprive A of his equal chance to avoid it and improve to a substantial degree just so that B can also achieve normality. But if A and B are moderately ill, the good of B's becoming normal could override A's claim to a chance. This possible implication comes close to a guarantee that we will focus on rescuing someone from a very bad fate if we can bring him up to a minimum level. Having done that, we will maximize outcome so as to produce normality where we can. Here is another implication. Suppose we could improve many moderately ill people a significant amount but not to normality by dividing a dose that would produce normality if given to one person. We should not divide the dose. (Here is an analogy with another domain—we can improve the artistic abilities of many people who are already moderately good at art to another level or we can invest in producing one great artist. We should do the latter, but not necessarily because we do a great deal of good for the person who becomes the great artist, but just because we produce a great artist.)

Whether or not we accept the mental-special view as presented, there is yet an additional factor to be considered in the case represented in figure 3.4. Having achieved normality, B may become self-sufficient, thus freeing up money to help A with clozapine as well. Then the issue becomes one of whether we require A to wait for B's recovery before undergoing treatment, losing his chance for earlier treatment. The answer may depend on how badly off each person is.

But now imagine another case. Suppose that with clozapine we can improve B's condition greatly and improve A's not very much. (We might imagine two different variations: [1] B is still not normal, and [2] B is normal. For present purposes, we need not worry about this distinction. I will not consider the possibility that we could make someone superior to normal. See figure 3.5.)

Even someone who rejects the mental-special view could believe that when the difference in mental condition that we can produce becomes quite great in this way, it may be morally appropriate to favor the person in whom we can produce more good, given that need and urgency are equal in both. This means that the greater concern with helping someone avoid a very bad fate than with providing additional improvements (and the recognition that each wants to be the one helped) does not imply that avoiding the worse fate is *all* we are con-

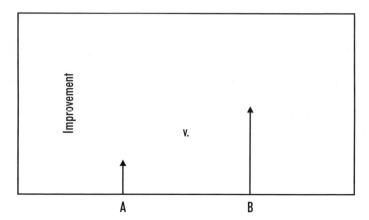

FIGURE 3.5   TWO-PERSON CHOICES: THE BELOW NORMAL CASE

cerned about. At least when we are also helping someone avoid the same very bad fate, our greater concern is combined with a lesser concern to produce additional significant improvement, and this may override concern for equal chances to avoid the very bad fate. However, the worse A's and B's conditions are in absolute terms without the drug the harder it is for extra good in B to overcome the claim that A has to an equal chance for significant improvement. The fact that the better A's and B's conditions are in absolute terms, the easier it is to override equal chances by a great good, makes this position close to a position guaranteeing requiring a chance at a minimum beyond which we can maximize, regardless of whether anyone achieves normality. (Notice that we can favor the person in whom we can produce much greater quality of life in non–life-and-death cases, even if the same sort of quality-of-life distinction is irrelevant in life-and-death cases.)

Let us change one of our assumptions and imagine that candidate B, but not A, is susceptible to moderate improvement with a drug other than clozapine—call it "mozapine"—that is inexpensive and not so scarce. Candidate B will not improve on mozapine as much as on clozapine, but he will improve as much as A would improve on clozapine. Suppose one of our principles is that we are more concerned with helping someone avoid a very bad fate than with providing additional improvement. Does this imply that we should make B ineligible to receive clozapine, for we can then treat both A and B, moving each away from a very bad fate? Not necessarily, for if we treat B with clozapine *and he attains normality* and self-sufficiency, he will be able to pay for his own maintenance on clozapine. We (i.e., public institutions) will then have money with which to treat A with clozapine as well. The trouble is that we may have to wait at least six months before we can treat A in this way, whereas if we keep B on mozapine, we can treat A right away. The question is whether some extra months of suffering on A's part are worth the goal of producing normality in B. The answer may vary depending on how bad A's condition is.

Helping More People

The last case again reminds us of the additional crucial factor in the clozapine case: more people can be helped if some rather than others are helped. Now, suppose that if and only if B is treated rather than A will money be freed up from his care so that someone else, C, can be treated as well. This is because only B achieves normality, and, once he does, it will be too late to treat A.

Suppose that all those who might be treated have the same need and urgency, and these are great. Then only if we treat B can we treat another person C who is as needy and urgent as A is (by hypothesis). This is a determinative reason for treating B rather than A, at least if the improvement in C is significant. But now suppose that we had to choose whether (1) to help B and C or (2) to help B and D, when C will improve to a moderate level but D will achieve normality. If money is freed up only if we help someone who becomes normal, and E (with the same need and urgency as A and a possibility for a significant outcome) is also waiting, then we should treat B and D rather than B and C (or A), for we can then treat E as well. (See figure 3.6.)

The principle that accounts for these judgments is that when need and urgency are constant, we ought to treat whoever allows us to treat as many people as possible, at least when the greater number of people will be helped significantly. Earlier, I argued that we should not always choose B over A when only these two people are in great need of help just because B will do better. Hence,

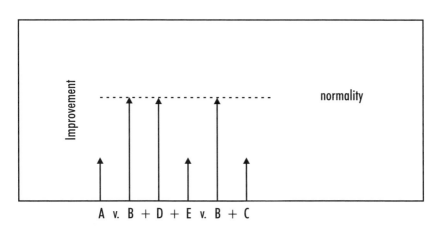

FIGURE 3.6   CASE OF MULTIPLE-PERSON CHOICES

if we should help B when other people's welfare is at stake, this implies that we are treating B as a means to the good of others, though not as a mere means since he also benefits.

Several objections can be raised to this analysis. The first objection is connected to the last point: The problem, it may be said, is not that we choose to help one person in part because this is a means to helping others. The problem is that the person who is *not helped* is evaluated solely from an instrumental point of view. (It might even be said that he is "treated as mere means," even though he is not causally useful in furthering our goal. This is because he is treated as a mere tool by being disposed of when he is not useful.) To make this clearer, consider the following example: If we face a choice between saving a doctor and a teacher, the fact that the doctor will be irreplaceable in saving lives should not mean that all the lives he will save (an indirect effect of the resource he gets) are counted on his side against the teacher. It might be suggested that this is true because the teacher who would not be selected for aid would be inappropriately evaluated from too instrumental a point of view, and not sufficiently as an end-in-himself. That is, it is only because he is *not* useful as a means in saving others that he is rejected for treatment. Is this not, it may be said, how the person who improves only moderately on clozapine is evaluated?

But now consider the following case: We have a scarce resource to distribute, and if we give it to A, he can then also carry it to another person, C, who needs our resource as much as A and B do. Person B cannot do this. In this case, it is permissible, I think, to select A over B, excluding B merely because he cannot be instrumentally useful. Doing this helps us to better serve those who directly need our resource. This contrasts with the previous case in which a doctor can save others who do not need our resource, but only need his skills. Hence (surprisingly), it is not distinguishing people on the basis of whether they have an instrumental role that determines if our behavior is objectionable, but rather whether our choice leads us to use our resource for its best *direct* (rather than indirect) effect. In the clozapine case, we select someone who will allow for the best direct use of our supply of clozapine, hence, the "treating as a mere means" objection does not defeat the strategy.[9]

A second objection to the analysis that allows us to help more people points to the difference between (a) denying someone treatment (either by not starting it, or by terminating a trial) in order to treat a greater number of other people *here and now*, and (b) denying someone treatment in order to treat a greater number of people *later*. Suppose we should give preference to the *here and now*. But, by hypothesis, we cannot treat B, D, and E simultaneously, for we must wait for B to recover in order for money to be freed up to treat D, and for the same reason we must wait for D to recover before we treat E. Theoretically, it could be a year before we get to helping E, if it takes six months for B and D to reach normality. Hence, here and now, it is a choice between A and B, and so, it might be said, we should toss a coin between them. However, even if we accept the correctness of giving preference to the here and now, we can answer this objection by noting that D and E do *here and now need to be treated*, even if we cannot treat them until later. Therefore, their case is different from the case of persons (statistically or even identifiable) whom we predict will need care in the future.

However, a third objection is waiting. We have assumed that we *know* that B and D will achieve normality, but in reality the problem is that we do not know who will achieve normality. So, at the time we must choose between A and B, we have no reason to believe that B will do better. Still, suppose we have already treated A for six months and he only improves moderately. Then there is at least a chance that B will achieve normality, but none that A will. If we drop A, we would do so in order to *go searching* for someone who will achieve normality so that we may help a greater number of people.

Therefore, even if numbers of those we can help matters morally, we must decide whether it matters more than (a) dropping someone after we have started treatment, in order to (b) only possibly help someone else more, in order to (c) only eventually help a greater number. I suggest that *at least when there is as yet no positive change in the patient's condition* (and so no regression*), the moral appropriateness of doing this depends on how long it will take to find someone who will achieve normality, and whether we are doing as much good in the interval as we would have done with the person dropped. Suppose that instead of six months, it took only one day to find out who would be normal (one day case). I suggest that objections arising from (a), (b), and (c) would then not be weighty, and we could morally afford to go searching for those who will allow us to treat the greater number. This suggests that what is problematic in the real case, where we must wait six months before we know if someone will be normal, is not (a), (b), or (c). Rather, it is (in addition to regression*) the possibility of a lengthy time during which no one is being helped who will increase the numbers helped as much as or more than A can.

But notice that what happens in one day in the one day case could be our *knowing* that someone will achieve normality, without his achieving it for six months. So we may still have to wait six months before treating someone else. When the *payoff* of treating more people is not achieved quickly, do factors (a), (b), and (c) loom large again? I suggest not. This implies that it is morally more important, at least when the person dropped has not yet improved, how long the gap is between dropping him and beginning treatment for someone else who will achieve normality, rather than how long the gap is between dropping him and treating a greater number of people.

What if A has already improved before we contemplate dropping him? Does the speed with which we can identify and begin treatment of someone who can become normal affect the permissibility of dropping A? If doing what leads to a patient's regression* is impermissible, the speed with which we find others to treat more successfully will not affect the impermissibility of dropping A. If regression* is not a barrier to helping a greater number of other people, the speed with which we can identify a candidate who will be normal and producing sufficient good should increase the permissibility of dropping someone.

Conflicts of Urgency and Outcome in Two-Person Choices

We have been assuming that all candidates for clozapine have the same need and urgency, and only varying outcomes. Now we come to deal with whether outcome dominates difference in severity. But degree of need and degree of urgency may themselves differ in the candidates. For example, there may be unequal need (as I have defined it) but equal urgency (as I have defined it). Suppose A is twenty years old, has had ten years of severe mental illness, and faces a bad future. Suppose B is twenty years old, has experienced moderate mental illness for the last year, and faces as bad a future as A. There is unequal need here, as A's life will have gone worse overall if he is not treated than B's life will have gone if he is not treated.

The type of case I wish to deal with in detail involves holding pasts equal, but varying urgency. How do we deal with differences in outcomes when some will be worse off than others if not treated (i.e., they are more urgent in my sense)? Let us start with two-person cases.

An easy case of this type is represented by figure 3.7, where "U" stands for urgency, "O" for outcome, and the numbers indicate the degree of each.

Here A is both more urgent *and* promises a better outcome (normality) if treated. Here there is no conflict between taking care of the person who would

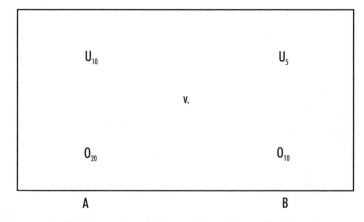

$$U_{10} \qquad\qquad U_5$$

v.

$$O_{20} \qquad\qquad O_{10}$$

A   B

FIGURE 3.7   CASE OF GREATER URGENCY AND OUTCOME COINCIDING

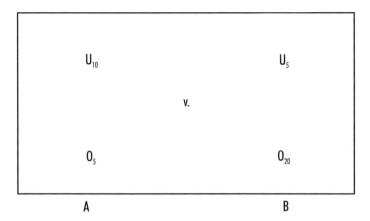

FIGURE 3.8 CASE OF GREATER URGENCY AND OUTCOME NOT COINCIDING

be worse off and treating the one who will produce the best outcome, at least if the difference in urgency between the two people is significant. But, of course, in another case, a conflict could arise between helping the person who would be worse off if not treated and producing the best outcome (normality). For example, see figure 3.8.

If U_{10} is a very bad prospect and O_5 is a significant outcome that lowers A's urgency to the level at which B is already, then it might be argued that we should first improve the condition of the worst-off person A, before producing a bigger benefit that goes to someone who is already better off. This conclusion follows from *maximin*, which is based on both a principle of fairness between people and the idea that we produce a morally more valuable outcome if we give even a smaller outcome to the worst-off person. This conclusion even follows from a nonmaximin principle, such as trying to bring those very badly off in an absolute sense to a minimal level, even if not always favoring the worst-off person.

An alternative position argues that we need not always favor the worst-off person, even when she is very badly off and we could make a significant improvement to a minimal level, if we can instead produce a much greater benefit in the life of someone else who is also badly off. According to this position, we should show that helping the worst off counts for somewhat more than merely producing the best outcome by assigning a factor with which we can multiply the outcome score of the worst off, in accord with the absolute (and relative) badness of her condition. This means we give the worst off an edge, but someone less badly off and with a better outcome could always win out. (Presumably, it would take a bigger outcome in the less urgent person to override the weight of urgency in the worst-off person by comparison to the outcome it takes in someone equally urgent to override the tendency to give the two equal chances.)

All these policies on how to deal with conflicts between urgency and outcome conflict with certain claims made about current clozapine policy.[10] For example, it is said that treating in accord with urgency and jeopardizing better outcomes is "against intuition." Policies I have described favoring worst-off individuals claim that it is not against intuition to do so. (Of course, given that urgency is no indication that clozapine will not lead to normality, sometimes there will be no conflict between favoring the urgent and producing the best outcome.)

It is also said that "no one argues against treatment when there is a dramatic response," that is, marked reduction of symptoms and restoration of normality. If this means that no one could reasonably argue against treating the most urgent who become normal, then that should be true. But if it means that no one could reasonably argue against treating those who would *not* be the worst off without treatment but who can achieve normality, then that is not true, at least in the two-person case.

Helping More People and Helping More Urgent People

Let us expand our conclusions about conflicts between urgency and outcome to deal with the additional crucial factor in the clozapine case, namely, that the number of people we can help may depend upon whom we help. Suppose A is more urgent than B but only B can achieve normality. (This assumes, hypothetically, that we could know before treatment who will become normal.) Suppose C is as urgent as A is and will produce as good an outcome. We free up money to help C only if we help B. So, should we help B and then C rather than A? (See figure 3.9.)

That choice seems peculiar. For if C is already in need now, why would we not choose to help him immediately? That is, why isn't it just a contest between A and C? The only answer available is that if we treat A or C first, we will never get to treat B, for A or C will not free up money for another patient. Here we are asked to consider letting a more severe patient suffer for some months while we treat a less severe patient simply because this allows us to treat both.

Suppose we can help B and C *or* B and D but not both sets. Patient D is as urgent as C (and A), but D and not C will achieve a normal outcome. Suppose E, who is as urgent as C, but cannot achieve normality, is also waiting to be treated. Only if we help D can we also help B and E, and so we should do this rather than helping B and C. We can then help two people who are as urgent as A instead of one person. (See figure 3.10.)

One way of interpreting the general principle at play here is as follows: Pay attention to best outcomes when doing so conflicts with taking care of the more

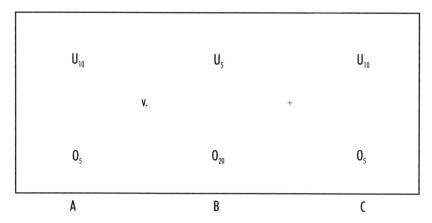

FIGURE 3.9   CASE OF HELPING MORE PEOPLE

urgent only if this makes it possible to significantly help more of those who are as urgent as those we might otherwise have helped. We do not so heavily favor those who give better outcomes per se; we favor them so heavily only when it helps us treat more who are urgent.

In the clozapine case, however, we are told that there will be no reason to think, at the time we make a choice, that someone as urgent as A will not have as good a chance of reaching normality as B and, hence, freeing up resources. It is also more important to treat the most urgent. Thus, it seems unlikely that it ever makes sense to treat the moderately ill B instead of someone more urgent.

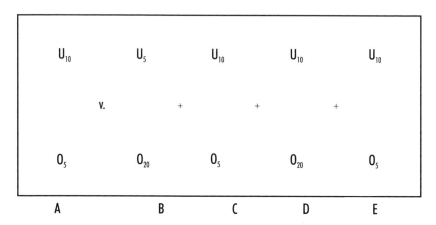

FIGURE 3.10   CASE OF PRODUCING MORE NORMAL PEOPLE

This means we should look for those who can produce normal outcomes among the urgent people only. (For one radical alternative to this, see the next section.)

Also, we cannot know that A will not produce a normal outcome until we treat for six months. On the basis of our previous discussion, we can see that two issues then arise. First, may we stop treating A after six months to test another urgent person for restored normality, or does regression* matter morally? Second, does it matter how long it is expected to take to find someone who will respond better than A and how much good we produce in the interval? On the assumption that there are now always additional urgent cases who could reach normality, and that it is not always wrong to stop or not start treating the most urgent who confront us, we should drop those who are urgent but have only moderate outcomes after six months of treatment, so as to search for those who are now urgent and who will achieve normality (as long as the probability of finding these is sufficiently high, and sufficient good is done in the interval of the search).

This policy, however, gives lexical priority to helping significantly as many of the worst-off individuals as we can. As noted earlier, an alternative is to give only somewhat greater weight to claims of the worst off or focus on them only if they are below a minimal state. On this alternative, we would not ignore the possibility of better outcomes in the less urgent or do whatever is necessary to maximize the number of most urgent people who get treated. This might mean also taking care of moderately ill people who will achieve normality in order to increase the number of people who achieve normality.

The Moderately Ill

If there were no more urgent cases to treat who could achieve normality, would a maximin policy say that those urgent individuals who could only achieve moderate outcomes should be favored over other patients who were already only moderately ill regardless of the outcomes that the latter would produce? If so, then concern for treating the worst off would come into real conflict with the desire to produce good outcomes and with the desire to treat as many patients as possible. For if we treated "moderates" rather than those "urgents" whom we know cannot achieve normality, we might achieve more cases of normality (albeit in those only moderately ill). However, if a policy of treating moderates who become normal freed up enough money to bring more urgents up to the level of moderate well-being in a reasonable time, we would get the benefits to moderates without too great a sacrifice to urgents. Even maximin could then recommend such a policy.

A radical alternative that opens up more possibilities for treating the moderately ill suggests itself. Consider that if we continue treating only those urgents who will become normal, they will wind up *better off* than those who were moderately ill to begin with. Out of fairness, we might stop fully treating the urgents at the point where they become moderately well—assuming we could maintain them at that degree of moderate well-being if full treatment did not continue— and then decide whether to bring them or those who had been already moderately ill (independent of clozapine) up to normality.

This proposal may strike many doctors as morally problematic: It would have them stop treatment although more good for a patient could be achieved. However, it is not problematic in the way regression* is, and I have already argued that commitment to one patient is not necessarily a strong enough consideration to override concern for other patients. Of course, in this situation, it is just a concern for fairness rather than better outcomes that is driving the proposal, since either patient (it is being hypothesized) could become normal.

A problem with this proposal is that we lose cost-effectiveness, for we use some of our clozapine resources to keep some people who would be urgent at the level of only moderate well-being. Those who survive at a moderate level without clozapine are costly because they require institutionalization, but they are not as costly as those who require institutionalization *and* also require clozapine treatment to achieve moderate well-being. Furthermore, when we partially treat a patient who could become normal to *search* for a moderate who could also be normal, we give up on a sure bet for many possible failures followed by a random choice.[11]

Notes

1. Other drugs may (or perhaps already have) come to supplant clozapine for treatment of schizophrenia. That will not affect the relevance of my discussion, because I take clozapine only as an example of a scarce resource. My discussion also applies to other scarce resources, such as places in intensive care units. However, the method I employ in this discussion may lead to different results where other scarce resources are involved because they do not share a particular characteristic assumed to be true of clozapine; the severely ill (what I call the most urgent cases) have as good a chance of attaining normality as those not already severely ill. In other situations (e.g., involving scarce organs for transplantation), severity of illness tends to be correlated with worse outcomes.

2. These are principles I have (for the most part) discussed in detail in my *Morality, Mortality*, vol. 1 (New York: Oxford University Press, 1993), and in the last part of my "Nonconsequentialism," in *The Blackwell Guide to Ethical Theory*, ed. Hugh LaFollette (Oxford: Blackwell Publishing, 1999).

3. In "Mental Health Services: Ethics of Resource Utilization" (unpublished: The Hastings Center, 1994).

4. I here make use of prospect theory developed by Daniel Kahneman and Amos Tversky. For more on this theory, see my "Moral Intuitions, Cognitive Psychology, and the Harming/Not Aiding Distinction," *Ethics* 108, no. 3 (April 1998).

5. See *Morality, Mortality*, vol. 1.

6. These claims are discussed in more detail in *Morality, Mortality*, vol. 1.

7. For reasons I will not go into here, I do not believe an *ex ante* perspective on the issue yields a different result.

8. Ruth Faden suggested something like this to me.

9. I first pointed this out in *Morality, Mortality*, vol. 1. I believe there is a striking similarity—indicating that the same underlying principle is at work—between what distinguishes the doctor and clozapine cases and what (I have elsewhere argued) distinguishes cases in which it is impermissible to favor using scarce resources on a nondisabled candidate rather than a disabled one from cases in which doing so is permissible. There, once again (I surmise), it turns out that we may favor a candidate whose makeup allows us to use our resources to do a better job but we may not favor a candidate who yields a better outcome simply by virtue of characteristics he brings to the situation. For more on this, see my "Disability, Discrimination, and Irrelevant Goods," (forthcoming in *Fairness and Goodness*, ed. D. Wickler, World Health Organization).

10. As reported in "Mental Health Services."

11. This essay was originally conceived in 1994 as a part of a Hastings Center Project on Mental Health. The version published here is only slightly modified from the version that previously appeared in *Medicine and Social Justice*, ed. Margaret Pabst Battin, Rosamund Rhodes, and Anita Silvers (New York: Oxford University Press, 2002). I am grateful for comments from members of the Hastings Center Project, from audiences at Stanford University Medical School and the Bioethics Institute at the Johns Hopkins University, and from Ruth Faden and John Oberdick.

CHAPTER 4

The Just Allocation of Mental Health Care

Eric Rakowski

HOW MUCH MENTAL health care should people generally have available to them? And how should that care be allocated if not everyone who might benefit from it can be helped? The answers to these questions depend primarily on the resolution of two more general issues. The first is a bedrock question of social justice: What principles ought to govern the distribution of resources and opportunities among a society's members, independent of any insurance decisions—with respect to health care, for example—they may legitimately make? The second issue concerns the limits to state paternalism. How much freedom should the government give people to risk or protect their physical or mental well-being? What costs should they bear if permissible gambles go awry or if they desire more security against ill health than a just scheme for allocating social resources necessarily affords them?

This essay begins by explaining why respect for individual autonomy implies that virtually all rights-based accounts of distributive justice, libertarian and egalitarian alike, agree on how health care should be distributed in most instances. In the majority of cases—those involving competent adults who are not known to face above-average, involuntary health risks—they all ground principles of allocation in the informed desires of competent insurance purchasers; independent moral principles play no part in distributing health care in these cases. Significant moral disagreements over how much health care children and those who are known to be genetically unlucky should receive at others' expense do exist among theories of distributive justice. But with respect to most privately insured individuals as well as most recipients of public assistance, the distribution of whatever quantity of care insurance premiums and tax dollars supply does not raise interesting moral questions, apart from those relating to collective decision making. The more important question for determining what care these people ought to receive is whether the state may compel them to do what it deems in their best interest when they do not share its view.

The balance of this essay explores the consequences of these abstract conclusions for the provision of mental health care within both private and publicly funded insurance plans. Its central claim is that resources should be devoted to treating those conditions that people who benefit from equal claims to health

79

insurance have or would have insured against before misfortune struck. The distribution of care should therefore typically depend on what people want or would have wanted by way of insurance, not on moral principles that refer to patients' comparative neediness. There are sound reasons for requiring people to insure against debilitating mental illness and a separate moral imperative to treat the severely and persistently mentally ill even if they cannot afford to pay. Because doctors and insurance administrators should be guided by patients' preferences in allocating care when resources are scant, however, they rarely face hard moral choices in deciding whom to help, outside of underfunded public assistance schemes targeted at people who are unjustly disadvantaged. The most difficult moral problems facing care providers are determining what manner of care people ought to receive if they never had a fair opportunity to insure and combining into one or a few insurance plans the conflicting preferences that people would come to have if they considered more carefully than consumers usually do the likely costs and benefits of available treatments.

Justice and Medical Need

Imagine a world in which property and opportunities are justly distributed. Imagine further that everyone is healthy and that nobody has any reason to think that her health or anyone else's health will decline. Now suppose that disease enters Eden, striking some but not all. Who ought to shoulder the cost of palliating or curing illness? Who should pay (if any other person should) to alleviate whatever added hardship somebody suffers if she is unable to work or enjoy life as she did before?

Personal Autonomy and Distributive Justice

Competing accounts of distributive justice offer a spectrum of responses to these questions. Some contend that, charity aside, losses ought to remain where they fall, regardless of how devastating they are. Thus a life marred by bad health yields no claim of justice against people who are luckier or richer; an unhealthy person might welcome help, but he has a right to assistance only if he insured beforehand.[1] A less grudging view finds in justice a safety net, woven to fit some notion of basic human needs or of proper sympathy for undeserved suffering. An adherent of this moderate position might claim that if somebody would be destitute if unaided, he is entitled to compensation from those spared his misfortune; however, if he could cope without severely impoverishing himself, then he must manage on his own. At the other edge of this rainbow are theories that regard people as obliged to share in one another's plight to a substantial degree. Utilitarianism offers one example. My theory of equality of fortune provides another, in holding that people disadvantaged through no fault of their own generally have a moral claim to help from those whom fortune blesses in order to restore as nearly as possible the fair footing on which they stood prior to the arbitrary onset of disease.[2]

For now, it is unimportant which of these theories is correct, for they share one vitally important feature. With the possible exception of utilitarianism and similar consequentialist approaches, which I shall ignore, these widely varying accounts of justice offer identical prescriptions for funding and delivering medical care in the majority of cases, notwithstanding their superficially divergent implications. More precisely, they agree about the health care entitlements of mentally competent adults who do not knowingly face higher-than-average health risks by virtue of genetic infirmities or other factors for which nobody can be held responsible.

Consider the view that unmerited inequalities ought to be extinguished (subject to constraints imposed by competing values), so that people stricken by cancer or schizophrenia are owed compensation by their luckier peers sufficient to put them as nearly as money and medical science can on the same plane of satisfaction and opportunity that they occupied before their health deteriorated. This view endorses what is tantamount to a mandatory insurance scheme in which each person receives exceedingly generous protection against adversity, at the price of being obliged to bankroll others if he evades sickness more successfully than they do.

However, if one believes that freedom of choice should be honored when it does no harm to others, an expensive insurance policy for all cannot be justified. People who wish to provide less assistance to those who turn out to have worse health should be free, if individual autonomy matters, to leave the insurance pool that justice initially prescribes. They may do so fairly if they agree, in the event that they are afflicted, to forego the assistance they would prefer not to supply to others. Their departure will not hurt those who elect to remain in the expensive insurance pool; those people will continue to receive the same protection they did before, at the same high price. No one will be worse off, and some will be better off, if people have the liberty to decide for themselves. Hence even a theory of justice that seems to require considerable redistribution to narrow any unearned material or experiential differences between people may embrace what amounts to a free market in insurance, so long as that theory prizes individual autonomy when one person's choices do not burden others. Indeed, all rights-based theories that respect personal autonomy will arrive at this conclusion, because any set of initial entitlements may be waived if people spy what they consider a better alternative.

The main differences between the leading nonconsequentialist theories of distributive justice therefore have nothing to do with their favoring or repudiating a health insurance market for rational adults who can shop on equal terms. They are manifest, instead, in their divergent views of the resources people ought to have available to them, with which they may or may not buy health insurance. The size of the disparities in people's initial entitlements profoundly influences how much health insurance they can and will buy, and it is their differing implications for income redistribution, and hence for health care distribution, that marks the largest divide between theories of justice.

These theories also part company in the way in which they cope with two classes of people: those who are known to face more serious health risks than others through no fault of their own, who would for that reason have to pay higher premiums in an unregulated market; and people who are not competent to buy insurance responsibly, such as children and the mentally ill.[3] The issues that these two classes present are closely aligned.

Unequal Risks That Are Known and Unmerited

One of the most basic disagreements among nonconsequentialist theories of justice is the provision they make for people who are disadvantaged through no fault of their own. If the disadvantage has not yet befallen an adult, or if it is unknown to him and others, the insurance market will charge him the same rates as it charges anybody else. There would be no injustice in leaving him to determine the breadth of his insurance coverage. What should be done, however, with regard to reasonable adults who are known to face abnormally high (or low) health risks on account of their genetic heritage or some childhood accident or illness?

Some notions of justice admit that these people are unlucky, because they must pay more for insurance than others do or must forego insurance altogether because none is offered to them, but these notions maintain that those people have no moral claim against those whom nature has favored. The view that others and I[4] share avers instead that justice requires evening out the effects of people's undeserved good or ill fortune insofar as that is practicable. Exactly how that should be accomplished is debatable, but any solution must substantially narrow the gap between the insurance rates faced by the fortunate and the unfortunate. The disparate approaches offered by competing theories of justice are reflected in current debates over national health insurance reform.

Youth and Mental Incompetence

Not everyone is a responsible adult whose possible health problems lie in the future and who must decide how much health insurance to buy in light of the risks he confronts. Many people are stricken before they have had a fair chance to insure. Some suffer from congenital disabilities or childhood mishaps or illnesses. Others never attain the mental competence necessary to make responsible health care decisions for themselves. What provision, if any, should be made for their medical misfortunes, given that they cannot be held responsible for not insuring against them?

This question poses, more starkly, the same issue as the preceding question about the unequal, undeserved risks that people are known to face. Two alternative responses seem to me especially attractive: the view that people who were unable to insure fairly should receive whatever assistance is needed to make up for their undeserved medical disadvantage, so long as transfers from the fortunate to the unfortunate yield substantial benefits to the latter without causing undue hardship to the more fortunate,[5] and Ronald Dworkin's view that compensation should be based on the insurance contracts that these people would have entered into had they been able to insure, where the best approximations of the terms of those hypothetical policies are extrapolations from the insurance decisions of competent adults.[6] Of course, many would not go as far as these two responses do. Some claim that justice mandates monetary transfers only to relieve the worst suffering of children and the mentally incompetent; a few see no need for any compensation at all. This debate will remain at the heart of Medicare reform in the United States.

Paternalism

One source of immense difference among approaches to distributing health care is independent of rival notions of justice. That source is incompatible ideas about the propriety of paternalism—of compelling people to act in a way that some authority believes is objectively in their best interest or is in accord with the decision they would have taken had they themselves known more or thought more carefully about what might happen to them.

The problem of paternalism is manifold. First, if paternalism is warranted, should it take the form of a requirement to purchase private insurance or of mandatory state-provided health care insurance? Second, according to what theory of individual self-interest or hypothetical choice should the scope of mandated health care be determined? This question calls for, at the least, an account of fully informed, rational deliberation given the aims an agent has at a given time; at the most, it requires an account of what is objectively prudent for someone and thus presupposes a theory of rationality toward the future stages of one's life.[7] The model of fully informed or rational choice that one selects crucially determines how much mental health care should be provided within private insurance plans and especially within government-run programs. On reflection, people might well choose to purchase less mental health insurance than experts familiar with mental health problems consider wise, and they might discount the value of their mental or physical well-being at some distant future time more than some philosophers believe is sensible. Third, if one accepts a full-information theory of prudence, rather than a stronger theory that finds a small set of health insurance plans prudent for everybody, one needs to say how people's diverse preferences are to be combined into one or a few health care plans, because greater variety would probably be impracticable. This is a difficult problem of democratic theory.

Intertwined with the question of paternalism is another: What moral obligations do individuals have to other members of their community to protect their own health, and may those obligations (if any) be enforced by the state? Must somebody get vaccinated, for example, to ensure that he does not contract some disease that he might spread to others? Is he obligated to buy at least minimal emergency medical insurance to avoid putting people in a position in which they must either pay for his care out of a sense of duty or altruism or let him die miserably? Should the government force him to buy insurance to prevent him from becoming a public charge?

My aim here is not to solve these problems but to suggest that philosophical and policy debates should focus on these questions. In the next section I describe several difficult moral issues that do *not* deserve attention in deciding how to distribute health care.

Moral Problems That Health Care Providers May Ignore

If one accepts one of the nonconsequentialist theories that respect individual autonomy (perhaps subject to paternalistic constraints), then several perplexing moral problems disappear when health care resources that are limited only by responsible adults' spending decisions are allocated.[8] One is the problem of fault. One might maintain that the blame somebody bears for her plight ought to determine where she stands in the line for medical care if some must be helped before others or whether she must pay for that care out of pocket. Using James Nelson's example,[9] one might assert that someone who was badly injured in an auto accident en route to a supermarket to buy something as trivial as potato chips or who develops cardiovascular disease because she ate too much fudge should have lower priority than somebody who suffers a like injury or disease doing something more socially useful or behaving more prudently.

This assertion might be true if medical assistance were offered as charity to the needy. But its correctness has no relevance to the distribution of medical care among responsible adults who have paid for their policies or who have equal claims to public assistance. It is for them as consumers to decide which eventualities they wish to insure against and in what way at whatever price the market charges. It is their preferences as insurance buyers, not the morality of their actions (except insofar as their moral convictions shape their insurance preferences), that determine what care they receive. They might very well choose to make fault a determinant of priority in some instances. If it becomes one, however, it is because people have decided to give it prominence, not because morality mandates that outcome.[10]

A second moral problem that vanishes in the case of competent adults is what Norman Daniels has called the "fair chances/best outcomes" problem.[11] Suppose that some medical treatment is in short supply because potential patients did not invest heavily enough to allow everyone to be helped when many people are simultaneously in need. Renal dialysis machines offer an example in some countries. If doctors must choose between two patients, one of whom will live longer or recover a higher level of functioning than the other, should they automatically favor the second? Should they instead take no account of the difference in outcomes and give both patients the same odds of receiving treatment? Or should they somehow acknowledge the value of both better results and fairness by conducting a lottery that gives more favorable odds to the patient who would benefit most from treatment?

In the absence of any insurance scheme, these choices would indeed pose difficult moral issues if doctors owned the resources that patients needed. If, however, responsible adults have an equal chance to buy health insurance or have an equal claim to public insurance, the choices that Daniels describes are morally unproblematic. The question is what advance arrangements people made when they insured. To be sure, some people buying insurance, or firms devising plans to appeal to insurance buyers, might find it hard to decide how they would like priority assigned in these situations. But there is no moral dimension to that choice if all can insure on equal terms. And most people would find the choice easy after consulting their self-interest: they would prefer policies that *ex ante* gave them the most years of life or that most improved their well-being.

Doctors generally face no moral dilemma in deciding to honor people's informed insurance choices; hence the fair chances/best outcomes problem is not a moral puzzle most need to resolve. Matters become more complicated, of course, if contract terms are unclear or there is reason to believe that people's insurance decisions were ill-considered or based on misinformation. The complication, however, is not that of determining the moral merits of favoring one patient over another. If rationing is unavoidable, the hard questions are what insurance terms people would have wanted had they pondered these choices more carefully and with better information and whether doctors should honor the preferences patients would have had if they conflict with preferences they did in fact express.[12]

The same analysis applies to a related moral issue, which Daniels terms the "aggregation" problem.[13] The aggregation problem is actually a combination of two separate moral problems. Its first half is the fair chances/best outcomes problem described earlier. Its second half is a numbers problem that parallels the fair chances/best outcomes problem. Suppose that you can provide the same individual benefit to each member of a small group of people or to each member of a larger group of different people. Should you help the larger group outright? Should you give each group the same chance of receiving the benefit? Or should you make odds proportional to group size? Daniels does not consider this numbers problem independently. Instead, his aggregation problem poses a narrower issue: if members of the smaller group would each receive a *bigger* benefit than would members of the larger group—more additional years of life, for example—how should we combine individual benefits and numbers in deciding whom to aid?[14]

In my view, the numbers problem, Daniels's aggregation problem, and other possible ways of combining the numbers and fair chances problems all dissolve within the framework I have described.[15] Difficult as these problems may be for a potential rescuer who happens on groups of people in need, who cannot save everybody with the resources he owns, and who is not bound by any convention or agreement with or among those in danger, these decisions should not pose complex moral problems for health care providers working within a system of private or public insurance if all patients have equally strong claims to protection. The allocation of health care ought to depend entirely on which precautions people have freely chosen to invest in (or would have chosen if in fact they made no explicit decision), provided that they were able to insure on equal terms and were not unjustly placed with respect to one another. Because they are deciding how to spend their own money or (in the case of people enrolled in public programs) dollars to which they have an equal claim, in a situation of equal ignorance regarding the future, no moral principle constrains their insurance decisions apart from any duties they owe to people whom they would burden should they fall seriously ill.

Thus several philosophers err, in my view, when they contend that the distribution of medical resources that are scarce owing to choice rather than nature should be governed by principles that give weight to randomness, differential outcomes, and other factors.[16] Perhaps people would choose those principles in making their insurance decisions, but there seems little reason to expect them to do so. If they acted in their self-interest in buying insurance, they would favor larger numbers and better individual results over randomness as rules for choosing recipients. Most important, no moral value compels them to decide according to some other rule. That is not to say that the decisions people face when purchasing health insurance are easy. Some are vexing, particularly if comparatively little is spent on insurance, because there is no obviously correct way to compare prudentially the value of various health improvements, let alone to weigh them against different numbers of years of additional life. The key point, however, is that the difficult questions these decisions raise are questions of rational choice, risk aversion, and the value of possible treatments, not of justice or of substantive morality except insofar as people have duties to themselves or those who are dependent on them.

Implications for Mental Health Care

What ramifications do these reflections have for the distribution of mental health care generally, and for Daniels's aggregation problem in particular? The remainder of this essay describes some major implications. I assume throughout that there is no reason of moral theory to treat mental and physical health problems differently.[17] Both are species of bad luck; if they impoverish an individual's life equally, they furnish the same right to redress. Competing theories of distributive justice disagree about how much (if any) right to compensation medical misfortune yields, but none distinguishes between physical dysfunction and setbacks to a person's sanity or emotional stability. The important question is not whether a person is laid low by mental or physical illness, to the extent that the two can be separated. It is rather whether uncourted misfortunes generate a right to assistance and, if they do, whether someone had a fair opportunity to defend against *any* threat to her well-being—medical or nonmedical—by avoiding a known risk or by buying insurance. For many egalitarian theories of justice, it is the distinction between those who lacked this chance and unlucky people who squandered their opportunity that undergirds the distinction between an unfortunate person's right to compensation and her plea for charity.

Private Mental Health Insurance

What provision should be made for mental disorders in private health insurance plans, *given* that long-term chronic conditions are covered—as they often are in the United States—by public health insurance? (I question the propriety of making chronic care a public responsibility later.) Leave aside for the moment the issue of whether insurance companies may charge higher rates or refuse coverage to people who are known to suffer from some mental disability or disease or who are known to be predisposed to one. The terms that private policies should contain turn primarily on whether paternalistic considerations justify compelling people to insure against mental illness, on how people's ideal preferences are best measured if they serve as the touchstone for insurance terms, and on how different people's divergent preferences ought to be aggregated in establishing insurance policies for sizable populations. Justice imposes no limitations whatever. This is plainly true if, as I believe, in a just world private insurance is best seen as an autonomy-respecting substitute for the more comprehensive insurance against misfortune that justice otherwise mandates. It is equally true, however, under any other theory of justice that allows autonomous individuals to waive their rights to compensation in return for relief from duties they consider onerous.

Does mental illness get short shrift in private health insurance plans today? It is hard to know. To offer a fair judgment, one would have to look carefully at the suffering and privation that patients with different illnesses endure, compare the benefits of treatments, and assess the trade-offs that plans actually make, which might be hard to measure because many treatment decisions are made at physicians' discretion, rather than according to clear rules laid down in advance. Rendering these judgments is a daunting task. I do not know enough about particular plans and the many medical conditions covered to venture specific or general conclusions. It should be clear, however, that restrictions on mental health coverage—limits on annual office visits, for example—are not necessarily unjust. Insured persons might want them, if they believe that patients are largely to blame for certain disorders or they do not trust doctors to limit care that is only marginally beneficial. Some of these beliefs might be misguided, and plan administrators may attempt to persuade insurance buyers that their views are mistaken. But surely people who insure of their own accord have the freedom to err.

Or do they? There are two main arguments for allowing the state to stipulate the terms of health insurance plans, including provisions governing mental health care. The first is that, left to themselves, people will make mistakes and harm themselves by not exercising sufficient foresight; the government should force them to behave prudently. The second argument is narrower. Many people who do not insure will unfairly burden their fellow citizens if their luck is bad, because it would be wrong to forsake them if they were in serious medical need and could not pay for essential treatment. Would-be risk takers may therefore be required to contribute in advance to the cost of the care they are likely to need later. This argument is narrower than the first because it applies only to medical care (including mental health care) that people *desperately* need but could not afford if they were not forced to insure; it does not extend to all the insurance that it would have been rational for someone to buy.

The first argument appears sound in theory, at least so far as insurance against the costs of treating mental illness is concerned. Many people may underestimate their chances of experiencing some mental reverse, whether because of the stigma that still attaches to mental illness or because they exaggerate the extent to which their mental and emotional stability lies within their control. But this first argument for paternalistic restraints on insurance rests on an assumption that, in practice, tends to undermine its theoretical cogency. It assumes that the government knows best what people genuinely, if unconsciously, want or need. Experience offers little reason to think, though, that letting fallible officials set the terms of private insurance contracts is likely to yield better results than letting fallible insurance buyers (or their more knowledgeable proxies) choose them instead. With reason, people might not want to entrust government officials with the responsibility of deciding how they should spend their insurance dollars. Moreover, unless the government required *everyone* to buy the mandated insurance, it would be unfair to force people who purchased private insurance to pay for specified protections when people who chose not to insure at all were exempt from this compulsion.

The second argument has more force, both theoretically and practically. If we have a duty to aid people who are badly in need, as I assume we do, we may prevent them from unjustly burdening us by triggering this duty. The obvious way to do so is to require that everyone insure against especially debilitating mental illness, even if they would not have done so on their own. It is important to bear in mind, however, that stipulating the terms of private insurance policies may not be the best solution. Governments could instead provide the necessary insurance—a health care safety net—and tax people to pay for it. Of course, that solution has its own shortcomings. Most important, it would forego the price restraints that competition allegedly brings. Perhaps a mandate that applied to all private insurance plans would be superior. Once again, though, if a mandate is to be fair, the government must extend it to everybody, not just those who presently buy health insurance. That seems unlikely to happen soon in the United States.

Preexisting Conditions

A sizable group of people who seek insurance against mental illness and its attendant costs, such as job loss or lowered earnings, would face higher than average rates or find it impossible to buy insurance if the market were the sole mechanism for obtaining insurance. Some of these people come from families with histories of mental illness and might reasonably be thought by insurers to be poorer risks; others show signs of mental illness in childhood or adolescence, before they enter the insurance market. In addition, people who have insured and who have experienced mental disorders as adults might find that their insurance rates would increase enormously if they were to change insurers. Should the law leave the market undisturbed?

My view is that it should not. Justice requires, I believe, that people who are set back through no fault of their own—as a result of genetic infirmity, congenital injury, or other misfortune for which they cannot fairly be deemed responsible—are entitled *at the very least* to insure against poor mental health on the same terms as everybody else; those who suffer from a young age, because illness struck before they could fairly decide which health risks to bear, are entitled *at the very least* to whatever compensation would be provided by the insurance policies that most competent people buy for themselves. I lack space to argue for that conception of justice here. But those who share my view that unmerited disadvantages in mental health ought to be alleviated insofar as compensation is effective and not unduly costly would condemn an insurance market that did not give special consideration to people disadvantaged by chance rather than human choice.

The solution is not to require all insurance firms to charge rates that are uninfluenced by the especially large costs that they expect certain insurance buyers to impose on them. That policy could unfairly disadvantage those insurance firms that are most competitive, if their low rates drew more than their proportionate share of people with high-cost debilities. A wiser choice would be a tax credit or an income tax deduction targeted at people who confront above-average insurance costs through no fault of their own, against the backdrop of a market setting rates according to differential risks.[18]

To be sure, this solution is hardly perfect. First, depending on the size of the credit or deduction, it would either fail to compensate blamelessly disadvantaged people fully or tempt insurers to pad their surcharges for these people, knowing that the government would pick up any price increase. Second, it would be hard, perhaps impossible, to distinguish people who bear no fault for their mental illness from those who do bear some responsibility or who failed to insure at the same rates as others when they had the chance and whose higher rates now flow from their earlier negligent insurance buying.

If one considers the government justified in forcing everyone to insure, by charging everyone for mandatory insurance through higher taxes, the second problem is insubstantial. By contrast, the first problem is real. We might very well have to choose between economic efficiency and complete compensation of all who deserve help. That we cannot achieve perfection, however, is a poor reason not to get as close as we can.

Chronic Mental Disorders: Who Should Pay?

There are three broad answers to the question of who should bear the costs of treating chronic mental illness. The first is that those who suffer should pay in full; if they failed to make adequate provision beforehand by buying suitable insurance (or working for an employer who provided insurance), then they must exhaust their savings or rely on private charity. The second answer is that the government ought to carry this burden by taxing people for the protection it provides. This amounts to universal insurance funded in whatever way the government determines people's tax bills. In the United States and most of Europe, this typically means that insurance costs would be a rising fraction of taxable income, though one can also imagine taxing people a fixed amount as a charge for identical insurance policies. The third possibility is for the government to mandate that private insurers include coverage for chronic mental health care as part of every health insurance policy they sell.

I believe that requiring people to buy health insurance against serious adversity is justified both paternalistically and as an essential means to prevent unlucky individuals from becoming dependent on people who cannot morally refuse to help them. Thus, the first answer will not do. People who suffer from severe and persistent mental illness should be treated, either through private health insurance plans constrained by law to provide coverage against chronic, serious mental illness or through a government-run universal insurance scheme. As for answers two and three, there is no essential difference between these alternative means for funding a basic insurance package against serious mental illness. There is, however, likely to be one contingent difference: public programs are apt to be funded by one of the major existing types of tax—an income or a property tax, most likely—which means that people would probably not pay equal premiums for equal coverage, as they would under private plans. This difference could in theory be eliminated by imposing an identical income tax surcharge on everyone (though that would not reach people who had no income to declare), but in practice some difference probably would exist. Efficiency concerns push in both directions: private insurers offer the benefits of competition, but government oversight to ensure that everybody enrolls in a private plan brings costs that a universal government program avoids.

Which approach ought to be adopted? In a world characterized by a just distribution of wealth and income, people ought to pay the same price for an insurance policy of equal value. Any departure from this rule would alter the just status quo. Either a public plan or mandatory private insurance terms would do, the decision hinging on the pertinent administrative and efficiency costs. A mandatory income tax surcharge, which could be avoided if a taxpayer provided proof that he had already obtained the prescribed mental health insurance privately, would be one possible solution.

In a world such as ours, marked by an unjust distribution of resources, the answer is less obvious. If the poor tend to be those who are treated most unjustly and who do not insure as frequently or as fully against mental illness, then insurance rates that discriminated in their favor—benefits that were funded by a progressive income tax, for example—would accomplish some redistribution and might advance rather than stymie justice. A system that consigned all chronic mental illness to the public sector, with the consequence that private insurance plans funded by a progressive income tax make exclusions for chronic conditions, would in that case also be a step in the right direction. Whether it would be a sufficiently large step depends on how unjust one deems the prevailing distribution of wealth and income and how far either possibility would go toward remedying what is offensive about the current regime. It might be that the most just system in the United States today would be one that requires people to insure privately if their income is above a set amount and that compels at least some of those people to pay taxes to provide mental (and physical) health coverage to those whose incomes fall below the threshold amount.

Public Mental Health Insurance

A wholly public, mandatory mental health insurance scheme would be consonant with virtually any rights-based theory of distributive justice paired with moderate paternalism, so long as the costs were properly apportioned. Considerations of administrability, efficiency, and personal autonomy, not considerations of justice, determine the choice between public and private plans.

Two questions of justice stand out with respect to public mental health programs. The first is how much money should be collected for this purpose (or for all forms of health care), who should be included in the class of recipients, and who should pay how much to fund this transfer. The second question is how money that is set aside for this purpose should be allocated among the class of recipients, whether or not the total sum is a just amount.

Let me focus on the second question. Assume that there is a fixed health care budget for a predetermined set of health care recipients. Assume further that each recipient has the same claim to health care services. Three issues then arise.

The first, and to my mind the hardest, is an issue I flagged earlier: how to determine what priority to give to people who blamelessly have suffered misfortune prior to their enrollment in this publicly funded insurance system. Those who have not yet suffered this kind of disadvantage when they become recipients of public assistance possess an equal claim to insurance, and a fortiori an equal claim to shape the terms of their collective insurance plan. But those who have already experienced bad luck in their health, such as children or adolescents who suffer from mental disorders, occupy a different position. The question with respect to them is whether one ought to extrapolate from the insurance preferences of people who have not experienced this adversity or whether they have a stronger claim to priority in treatment than most people would choose to insure for.

The second and third issues are closely related and have already been stated. How are we to determine what insurance terms the recipients of public assistance would choose if they were better informed and acted prudently? And if they would disagree, because some infirmities seem to some people more dreadful than they seem to others and some possible treatments are in their view more worthwhile than other people believe them to be, how are their preferences to be combined in establishing a single public plan?

In practice, the third issue seems likely to dissolve into the second. Even if public opinion is canvassed with care, as Oregon did in devising its plan for allocating public health care dollars, the final decision will almost inevitably reflect the carefully considered preferences of experts who are more familiar with possible condition-treatment pairs than members of the covered public and who perhaps strive harder to achieve consistency in their allocation decisions than would respondents to opinion polls. A small group of experts is likely to have less diversity of viewpoint than a broad swathe of the uninformed public. Therefore, the third issue may have small practical significance. What deserves emphasis, once again, is that this expert-driven process of determining what insurance people would have purchased, trying though it is, does not entail controversial moral judgments. The hard judgments that it calls on insurance buyers to make are self-interested judgments about risk taking and the value of possible futures. The only difficult moral judgment, if health care resources are not naturally limited (as transplant organs are), is whether to give special consideration to people who were disadvantaged before they had an opportunity to protect themselves by acting responsibly or by insuring on their own.

Bipolar Patients and the Aggregation Problem

Bentson McFarland's case study, presented in chapter 5 of this volume, helpfully captures the multiple uncertainties besetting a clinician in a health maintenance organization. As he notes, a doctor's decision regarding whom to help may be clouded by the ambiguous terms of health insurance contracts, by the precarious availability of possibly unsatisfactory long-term care through publicly funded programs, by uncertainty about the consequences of treating one patient before another, and by the difficulty of accurately diagnosing patients' conditions, which affects who provides and pays for care and how the queue within a health maintenance organization is arranged. McFarland's illustration of Daniels's aggregation problem, however, abstracts from these uncertainties, at least as I understand it. I take his question to be this: If a clinician must decide to help one bipolar patient, five unipolar depressed patients, or ten patients suffering from panic disorder, how should she spend her time?

I cannot offer anything approaching a complete answer to this question. My hope (and expectation) is that under virtually all actual insurance plans, each of these people would receive adequate treatment. But even granting McFarland's assumption that choice is unavoidable, I find his question difficult to answer because I do not know just how terrible the suffering associated with each of these conditions is or how perilous they are. I also do not know whether it is possible to provide suboptimal treatment to all five of the depressed patients and all or most of the ten panic disorder patients, with results that the group of fifteen would prefer to the results of treating only the five or only the ten if the fifteen had to choose a course of treatment beforehand, not knowing whether they will be among the five or the ten. If the reasoning of this essay is sound, however, it is not difficult to state the proper approach to the question McFarland poses if one assumes that his clinician can treat only one of the three groups of patients.

It appears from his description that chronic patients are covered by a public mental health program and that the health maintenance organization contract was drafted to exclude long-term care precisely because it was available elsewhere. If so, then McFarland's clinician should send bipolar patients who need long-term treatment to that program. It might, as he notes, be difficult to diagnose bipolar disorder in some patients, but once a diagnosis has been reasonably established, the right decision is plain, especially given the hypothetical clinician's stretched resources. Nor is a system that consigns long-term care to public programs while leaving short-term care to private arrangements in any way immoral. One can easily imagine a just community dividing responsibilities in this way, requiring in effect mandatory catastrophic illness insurance under government auspices and permitting private insurance arrangements to supplement that care. To the extent that one finds the current system inequitable, as I do and as McFarland appears to do, one's objection must be to the underlying distribution of wealth and income, not to the assignment to different insurance plans of long-term and short-term care.

As to the choice between the five unipolar depressed patients and the ten suffering from panic disorder (or the one bipolar patient if no public program will take her), the relevant question is what treatment policy these patients would themselves have wanted if they were earlier asked to choose how to allocate the physician's time, in ignorance of their fate but in full awareness of what differences the two options would make to the lives of those who received treatment and those who did not. That might be a hard judgment for a physician to make, just as it would be a hard decision for someone selecting insurance terms. Perhaps in a just world it would never have to be made, because ample resources ordinarily would be available to treat all needy patients. But in our world it is sometimes inescapable, and the only fair way to decide is by appealing to what was, or what would have been, the free choice of those who are subject to the policy. Ideally, insurers would issue guidelines to physicians covering anticipated trade-offs of this kind. In their absence, however, the clinician McFarland describes would herself have to speculate as to what patients' antecedent, informed preferences would be.

A clinician might find this advice meager, preferring instead a rule that reduces her discretion or the complexity of the judgment she faces. That longing would be understandable. Because we cannot (or, at any rate, do not) write rules to cover every treatment decision in advance, however, I see no way to ease her predicament.

Notes

1. Jan Narveson, *The Libertarian Idea* (Philadelphia: Temple University Press, 1988), 245–68; Robert Nozick, *Anarchy, State, and Utopia* (New York: Basic Books, 1974), 213–31.

2. Eric Rakowski, *Equal Justice* (Oxford: Oxford University Press, 1991), 73–76, 88–92.

3. These theories also disagree about cases in which the scarce medical resource is limited by nature rather than by patients' earlier decisions not to create more of the resource. If two patients, ages thirty and sixty, each need a kidney to survive or to enjoy a higher-quality life, should they be allowed to bid for the one available organ in an auction? Should potential donors be permitted to sell, while alive, a kidney to

either? Disagreement abounds as well over who should control the disposition of transplantable cadaver organs. The state, because cadaver organs are a collective resource? The decedent, if she made prior provision? The decedent's heirs or assigns? I offer tentative answers in Rakowski, *Equal Justice*, 167–95, 324–31.

4. See, e.g., G. A. Cohen, "On the Currency of Egalitarian Justice," *Ethics* 99, no. 4 (1989): 906–44, at 916–21; Amartya Sen, "Capability and Well-Being," in *The Quality of Life*, ed. Martha C. Nussbaum and Amartya Sen (Oxford: Oxford University Press, 1993), 30–53.

5. Rakowski, *Equal Justice*, 92–106.

6. Ronald Dworkin, "What Is Equality? Part 2: Equality of Resources," *Philosophy and Public Affairs* 10 (1981): 283–345, at 298–304.

7. Helpful sources include Joel Feinberg, *Harm to Self* (New York: Oxford University Press, 1986); Donald VanDeVeer, *Paternalistic Intervention* (Princeton, N.J.: Princeton University Press, 1986); Rolf Sartorius, ed., *Paternalism* (Minneapolis: University of Minnesota Press, 1983); Connie S. Rosati, "Persons, Perspectives, and Full Information Accounts of the Good," *Ethics* 105 (1995): 296–325; Danny Scoccia, "Paternalism and Respect for Autonomy," *Ethics* 100 (1990): 318–34; Dan W. Brock, "Paternalism and Autonomy," *Ethics* 98 (1988): 550–65; Douglas N. Husak, "Paternalism and Autonomy," *Philosophy and Public Affairs* 10 (1980): 27–46.

8. I assume that the only paternalistic constraints that may be appropriate are those that would promote an individual's *nonmoral* welfare over time. If those constraints were instead designed to ensure that an individual acted with a proper moral regard for others in buying health insurance, then the moral problems I describe in this section would disappear, only to resurface within the theory of paternalism. I reject the view that they have a place there.

9. James Lindemann Nelson, "Publicity and Pricelessness: Grassroots Decisionmaking and Justice in Rationing," *Journal of Medicine and Philosophy* 19 (1994): 333–42, at 339.

10. The market might fail to make all the distinctions and exclusions that a particular person wants, because in practice there is some limit to how many policies an insurer can offer. There is, however, no injustice in this result. People would overwhelmingly favor a market solution to a long list of government mandated health care options that allowed them to tailor policies more snugly to their preferences. If providing those options at high cost were efficient, insurance companies would probably offer them; the fact that they are unavailable is strong evidence that the cost of offering more options is higher than most people believe that more exact tailoring is worth.

11. Norman Daniels, "Four Unsolved Rationing Problems: A Challenge," *Hastings Center Report* 24, no. 4 (1994): 27–29, at 27.

12. I describe the moral force of hypothetical rational consent in Eric Rakowski, "Taking and Saving Lives," *Columbia Law Review* 93 (1993): 1063–1156, at 1107–41.

13. Daniels, "Four Unsolved Rationing Problems," 28.

14. There are other aggregation problems that Daniels does not mention. What if members of the larger group would each receive a *larger* benefit than would members of

the smaller group? Should randomness be the rule in the face, simultaneously, of greater numbers and greater individual benefits? Or what if the larger group contains the one person who would benefit most and many others who would benefit very little, whereas the smaller group contains people who would all benefit substantially, yet each would benefit less than the anomalous member of the larger group?

15. For a more detailed statement of this argument, see Eric Rakowski, "The Aggregation Problem," *Hastings Center Report* 24, no. 4 (1994): 33–36.

16. Frances M. Kamm, "To Whom?" *Hastings Center Report* 24, no. 4 (1994):29–32, at 31–32; John Broome, "Selecting People Randomly," *Ethics* 95 (1984): 38–55; Michael Lockwood, "Quality of Life and Resource Allocation," in *Philosophy and Medical Welfare*, ed. J. M. Bell and Susan Mendus (Cambridge: Cambridge University Press, 1988), 33–55, at 54.

17. Philip J. Boyle and Daniel Callahan, "Minds and Hearts: Priorities in Mental Health Services," special supplement, *Hastings Center Report* 23, no. 5 (1993): S1–S23, at S11.

18. Rakowski, *Equal Justice*, 90–92.

CHAPTER 5

Resource Allocation for Mental Health Care and the Aggregation Problem

Bentson H. McFarland

RESOURCE ALLOCATION FOR mental health care raises a number of ethical considerations.[1] One such issue is what Norman Daniels[2] has called the aggregation problem. Clinicians working in systems with limited resources deal with the aggregation problem daily when they decide whether to spend an hour working with a single severely ill person or to use the same amount of time to serve three less ill individuals.[3] The rapid growth of prepaid (capitated) health care[4] has stimulated discussion about providing health care (and mental health care) to a defined population while operating under a fixed budget. In effect, capitation implies that resources provided to one individual will not be available for someone else. Using other terminology, the size of the pie has been fixed and the question is whether to give a large slice to one person or small slices to several other people.

Case Examples

Clinical case examples will make this point clearer. Bipolar disorder (also known as manic depressive illness) is a biologically based brain disease characterized by episodes of severely disabling mental illness separated by months, years, or decades of normal functioning. By definition, bipolar patients have experienced at least one episode of mania—a condition characterized by weeks of elevated mood, lack of sleep, poor judgment, irritability, or grandiosity that often results in hospitalization.[5] Most people with bipolar disorder also have episodes of depression characterized by low mood, lack of enjoyment, suicidal ideation, and difficulty with sleep or appetite among other problems. Bipolar disorder affects about one percent of the population and typically begins in adolescence or early adulthood. Heredity appears involved in most cases of the condition. It is important to distinguish between bipolar disorder and the much more common unipolar major depressive disorder. Persons with unipolar depression, by definition, do not have manic episodes.

Many patients with bipolar disorder respond to prophylactic medications and, for the most part, lead normal lives.[6] On the other hand, a significant number either fail to respond to treatment or decline to adhere to therapy with subsequent deterioration in their clinical condition. Early in the course of the illness it can be difficult to predict whether a patient with bipolar disorder will be "high" versus "low" functioning. There is some evidence to suggest that early and consistent treatment with medication can minimize one's chances of deterioration.[7]

Health maintenance organizations (HMOs) are prepaid managed care systems whose clinicians are obliged to provide enrollees with those services believed to be "medically necessary." Typical contracts between an HMO and a payer will state that medical necessity is determined by the HMO's clinicians.[8] Contract language for mental health often limits the HMO's responsibility to the treatment of conditions that the attending physician believes will resolve with relatively short-term therapy. The implication is that enrollees with chronic conditions will be served by the public mental health system. Interestingly enough, it is not uncommon for HMO members to find themselves referred back to the HMO by the public program (for at least some components of mental health care).

In staff and group model HMOs, mental health clinicians are usually salaried employees. Resources within the HMO's mental health department are, essentially, hours of clinician time. An hour devoted to one patient is an hour taken from another patient. Spending time with established patients means (potentially) that new patients must remain longer on the waiting list.

The clinician who authorizes treatment within the HMO for a bipolar patient may be committing the organization to deliver dozens of hours of outpatient service annually (not to mention the possibility of inpatient care). These hours might, for example, be psychiatrist time needed for the adjustment of medications. Those same hours could be devoted to seeing several patients with more benign conditions such as anxiety or unipolar depression. The HMO psychiatrist, for example, could provide medication evaluations and consultations to primary care providers for several panic disorder patients in the time that would have been devoted to a single (low functioning) bipolar patient.

A related problem is the flow of patients through the HMO's mental health department. Typically, HMO mental health clinicians will be presented each day with one or two new patients. The implication here is that (other things being equal) treatment for established patients must be discontinued at about the same rate. A "high functioning" bipolar patient may need relatively little mental health treatment (especially if the person's medications can be managed by a primary care provider). Conversely, the "low functioning" bipolar patient may require intensive specialty mental health care indefinitely.

On the other hand, the HMO clinician who invokes the "short-term therapy" condition and denies services may be sending the bipolar patient to an uncertain fate in a fragmented public mental health system. This issue, not surprisingly, has stimulated considerable debate and some litigation.[9]

The aggregation problem facing an HMO triage clinician, then, is how to balance the needs of one (low functioning) bipolar patient against, say, five (unipolar) depressed patients or perhaps ten panic disorder patients. In general, these conditions vary in the extent of associated disability. Panic disorder, for example, is characterized by spontaneous episodes of rapid heartbeat, quick breathing, sweating, tremors, and fears of impending doom.[10] The condition is very uncomfortable and often prompts patients to visit the emergency room. On the other hand, panic disorder, per se, is not fatal (although a third of persons with panic disorder have comorbid depression). Conversely, depression and bipolar disorder are associated with high rates of death by suicide.

At first glance, it might appear straightforward to invoke the short-term therapy contract language and deny services to bipolar patients. Clinicians dealing with an adolescent having her first psychiatric hospitalization can find the situation a bit more complicated. Because there are (at the moment) no laboratory tests or x-ray studies that can "prove" the presence (or absence) of bipolar disorder, the key to diagnosis is the clinical course. The implication here is that a condition originally thought to be mania might, in retrospect, turn out to have been an episode of stimulant drug abuse. Treatment of chemical dependency problems is usually a covered benefit in most HMOs. Even if the patient's condition is bipolar disorder, the long-term course can be difficult to predict. From an ethical perspective, of course, invoking the short-term therapy contract language simply transfers the resource allocation problem out of the HMO and into the public sector. Indeed, legislation in some states appears to nullify the short-term therapy contract language (at least for "biologically based" mental conditions such as bipolar disorder).

David Mechanic[11] feels that these questions of health care rationing should be dealt with in an "implicit" fashion and worked out on a micro level among patients and clinicians. The argument is that an explicit rationing system is difficult if not impossible to implement in present-day society. Wendy Mariner[12] distinguishes among "macro-allocation" (e.g., resources assigned to health care as opposed to education or transportation), "micro-allocation" (e.g., health care resources assigned to mental health as opposed to dermatology or cardiology), and "rationing" (when an individual patient is denied a health care service that might possibly be beneficial). She argues that rationing may not be possible in the United States until people are convinced that there is a true scarcity of health care resources at the macro level.

Taking another approach, Eric Rakowski[13] addresses these issues by focusing on the health insurance contract. In effect, Rakowski says that providers are ethically obliged to adhere to the terms of the contract. The notion here is that individual autonomy is best respected by making use of the insurance mechanism. People choose what sort of care they want when they make decisions about health insurance. As we shall see, this approach has certain features that are theoretically attractive but may be difficult to implement.

Maximum Autonomy Model

It is useful to begin the analysis by considering an idealized and greatly simplified situation that provides "maximum autonomy" health insurance. Here we assume that consumers can choose whatever health insurance they wish. We ignore (for the moment) the problems Rakowski mentions with regard to children, incompetent adults, the poor, and the chronically ill. We address these latter issues when we discuss the "limited autonomy" health insurance model.

Important features of the maximum autonomy health insurance model include availability of insurance, excludability of health services, and adequacy of information. These components are, in fact, required to make the system operate as proposed by Rakowski. First, health insurance must obviously be available for purchase by consumers. More to the point, there must be available a wide array of policies with different benefit structures. In order to maximize autonomy, people need to purchase the precise type of insurance that satisfies their individual desires. Further, these assorted insurance contracts must be renegotiated frequently (e.g., annually) to take account of changes in people's desires. A person's desire for health insurance coverage might well change due to aging, new family relationships, advances in medical technology, and the like. In the maximum autonomy model, it is assumed that the marketplace can generate this vast array of "tailor made" insurance policies and that they can be updated frequently.

One can wonder whether or not such an insurance marketplace could, in fact, be made to function. Consider, for example, the problem of pricing the policies. In a situation where a policy might be held by only one subscriber, how will the insurer get the data needed to set the price? Insurance pricing depends on the generation of claims by a population of covered lives sufficiently large as to reduce chance fluctuations to an acceptable level. There may be substantial actuarial problems in pricing insurance policies that are tailored for a small number of people. Another pricing problem relates to the notion of "moral hazard."[14] In other words, those who are well insured may be tempted to demand desirable but not medically necessary services (such as cosmetic surgery, psychoanalysis, and so on). Again, the insurer is faced with the challenge of pricing policies that might generate unlimited claims. However, if the "tailor-made" policy is replaced by a "standard" policy, then autonomy becomes less than maximal. Of course, insurers could offer tailor-made policies, but with exorbitant premiums.

Second, the maximum autonomy system would require the redefinition of health services as "excludable" goods. Here an excludable good is one that can be denied to those who are not able to pay for it.[15] In this context, health care would be provided only to the insured (or, presumably, to those able to pay out of pocket). Remembering that for the moment we have suppressed concerns about poverty preventing the purchase of health care, the rule would be "no insurance, no service."

The rationale here is threefold. First, the provision of care to uninsured people would in this system mean that services were less available to the insured, which appears to be both unethical and a violation of contracts. Second, there would be no incentive to insure oneself if uncompensated care were readily available. Third, providers need to know consumers' desires (if any) for health care. Those who elect not to be insured are also declining future health services. The maximum autonomy system requires people to make decisions about health insurance.

In this system, then, the provider would have to adopt an attitude of "you made your bed and now you must lie (or, more to the point, perhaps die) in it." Obviously, this hard-nosed attitude to those who are voluntarily uninsured represents a substantial change in traditional, paternalistic medical ethics. However, Robert George and I have pointed out that clinicians are already shifting their focus away from the individual patient and toward the larger population.[16] Although it sounds farfetched, the "no insurance, no service" system might simply be (for better or worse) the culmination of an ongoing trend.

Finally, consumers operating in a maximum autonomy system need sufficient information to make rational choices. Obviously, people would have to appreciate the "no insurance, no service" rule. Perhaps more important, though, is the need for people to insure themselves against unlikely but potentially devastating events. For example, 99 percent of people will not have bipolar disorder, but it is well known that 1 percent of the population will develop this condition. Consumers would need education about decision making under uncertainty.

Although it is generally believed that people tend to underinsure with respect to mental illness, there is a suggestion from work by David Pollack and his colleagues[17] that consumers can be educated about the severity and treatability of mental disorders. The authors noted that in the Oregon approach to prioritizing health services, people did rank mental illnesses high in the list of conditions meriting treatment once they had learned about these disorders.

Indeed, the maximum autonomy approach might require considerable work on the part of consumers who would need to specify what sorts of treatments (if any) they desire. Of course, consumers could (as now) purchase policies entitling them to medically necessary care. However, as the case examples pointed out, much of our current difficulty in health care resource allocation revolves around the definition of medical necessity.[18]

Assuming that these implementation problems could be solved, the maximum autonomy model would neatly address the issue of resource allocation. The size of the health care pie would be determined by the premiums paid for health insurance. The division of the pie into its various sectors (physical health, mental health, etc.) would be determined by the wording of the assorted health insurance policies currently in force. Consumers would be entitled to what they specified in their tailor-made health insurance policy (but no more). As noted, however, the maximum autonomy approach would require substantial (indeed overwhelming) behavior change in markets, providers, and consumers. Furthermore, we have until now neglected the issues raised by children, incompetent adults, the poor, and the chronically ill. In addition, we will need to return to the "voluntarily uninsured."

Limited Autonomy Model

Rakowski points out that considerable modification must be made if what I have termed the maximum autonomy model is to function in the real world. Obviously, some people are by definition not autonomous consumers. Children (and incompetent adults) cannot be expected to make complex health insurance purchasing decisions. Ideally, parents or guardians would be able to select the appropriate health insurance. But what if these proxy consumers are not available (or do not act in the best interest of the child or the incompetent adult)? What about people too poor to afford any health insurance or unable to afford the tailor-made coverage they would prefer? This last group could well include the medically indigent who are unable to afford coverage due to preexisting (typically chronic) medical conditions. One suggestion is to provide such individuals with the health insurance they would have purchased had they been able to do so.

As always in health care, the devil really is in the details. How exactly will we determine what health insurance coverage (among the large universe of tailor-made policies) the individual would have purchased? For children or incompetent adults, one could claim that the appropriate choice is the most common type of policy in the absence of better information. One could also use the person's demographic characteristics (age, gender, residence, etc.) and try to predict what policy she would have chosen (based on data from the insured population). One might even try to use medical history data in an attempt to improve the accuracy of prediction. For the poor or the medically indigent, one could provide the individual with the policy that he or she would have selected had sufficient funds been available.

The next logical question is who will pay for this coverage. Presumably society (via a government mechanism) will purchase insurance for these people. Inconveniently, voters' apathy toward new tax burdens[19] suggests that the government (at least in the United States) is unlikely to finance high-cost insurance for this population. If Oregon's tumultuous debate about health care for the uninsured is any example, the insurance coverage will be "basic" indeed.[20] Taxpayers, voters, and their elected representatives appear to have little interest in maximizing autonomy for the uninsured.

We are left then with the task of defining basic health care. In the process of doing so we are ipso facto indicating the amount of resources we are willing to allocate for the provision of these services to people who are (for whatever reason) unable to participate as consumers in the health insurance marketplace.

Similar considerations apply to the voluntary uninsured. Rakowski[21] suggests that government could provide "a health care safety net" financed by taxes. Feldstein[22] has proposed that income-related vouchers be made available for purchase of health insurance. Presumably, the voucher or the safety net would translate into basic health care insurance coverage. As Rakowski notes, such an approach to universal health insurance appears unlikely to happen soon in the United States. Nonetheless there is value in addressing the ethical implications of such a system.

First, it is clear that the health care safety net approach represents a reduction in personal autonomy. Individuals would not be allowed to go without health insurance. Perhaps more important, children, incompetent adults, the poor, and the medically indigent would be restricted to the safety net with a consequent diminution in autonomy. This system, then, is a limited autonomy model.

Second, the introduction of the safety net has important implications for the marketplace in health insurance—namely, there is now a problem of adverse selection.[23] Those who are healthy might well be satisfied with the safety net's insurance coverage, whereas those who are ill (but not medically indigent) might elect to stay in the insurance marketplace. Consequently there could be an acceleration of claims in the commercially insured population while the safety net system acquires healthier enrollees. Also, employers may be tempted to discontinue the provision of health insurance, knowing that the safety net is available.

Finally, the limited autonomy system does not address the resource allocation problem in such a tidy way as did the maximum autonomy approach. Given that the safety net will provide insurance for a large (and perhaps growing) fraction of the population, then we have simply transferred the concerns about allocation of resources and aggregation of individuals to the safety net enrollees. We have, unfortunately, come full circle.

Respecting individual autonomy through the use of insurance can theoretically address several challenges of health care rationing, including the aggregation problem. However, implementing in the real world a system designed to maximize autonomy raises numerous difficulties. When the health insurance system is modified so as to limit autonomy but ease implementation, the rationing problems (including aggregation) reemerge.

Notes

1. Philip J. Boyle and Daniel Callahan, "Managed Care in Mental Health: The Ethical Issues," *Health Affairs* 14 (1995): 7–22; Robert A. George et al., "Managed Care and Health Care Rationing," *Child and Adolescent Psychiatric Clinics of North America* 4 (1995): 869–83.

2. Norman Daniels, "Four Unresolved Rationing Problems: A Challenge," *Hastings Center Report* 24 (1994): 27–29.

3. Bentson H. McFarland and Robert A. George, "Ethics and Managed Care," *Child and Adolescent Psychiatric Clinics of North America* 4 (October 1995): 885–901.

4. Bentson H. McFarland, "Health Maintenance Organizations and Persons with Severe Mental Illness," *Community Mental Health Journal* 30 (1994): 221–42.

5. American Psychiatric Association, *Diagnostic and Statistical Manual of Mental Disorders*, 4th ed. (Washington, D.C.: APA 1994).

6. American Psychiatric Association, *Practice Guidelines for the Treatment of Patients with Bipolar Disorder*, rev. ed. (Washington, D.C.: APA 2002).

7. Ibid.

8. McFarland and George, "Ethics and Managed Care," 885–901.

9. Ibid.

10. American Psychiatric Association, *Diagnostic and Statistical Manual*.

11. David Mechanic, "Dilemmas in Rationing Health Care Services: The Case for Implicit Rationing," *British Medical Journal* 310 (1995): 1655–59.

12. W. K. Mariner, "Rationing Health Care and the Need for Credible Scarcity: Why Americans Can't Say No," *American Journal of Public Health* 85 (1995): 1439–45.

13. See Eric Rakowski, "The Just Allocation of Mental Health Care," chapter 4 of this book.

14. P. J. Feldstein, *Health Care Economics*, 4th ed. (Albany, N.Y.: Delmar Publishers, 1993).

15. W. Baumol and A. S. Blinder, *Macroeconomics: Principles and Policy* (Fort Worth, Tex.: Dryden Press, 1994).

16. McFarland and George, "Ethics and Managed Care."

17. David A. Pollack et al., "The Prioritization of Mental Health Services in Oregon," in *What Price Mental Health? The Ethics and Politics of Setting Priorities*, ed. Philip J. Boyle and Daniel Callahan (Washington, D.C.: Georgetown University Press, 1995).
18. McFarland and George, "Ethics and Managed Care."
19. Mechanic, "Dilemmas in Rationing."
20. Pollack et al., "Prioritization of Mental Health."
21. Rakowski, "Just Allocation of Mental Health Care," chapter 4 of this book.
22. Feldstein, *Health Care Economics*.
23. Ibid.

CHAPTER 6

Autonomy, Reality, and the Just Allocation of Mental Health Care

Laura Weiss Roberts, Teresita McCarty, and Sally K. Severino

> *The difficulty in life is the choice.*
> —George Moore

> *Justice is the hope of all who suffer.*
> —John Greenleaf Whittier

AUTONOMY AND FAIRNESS are two principles guiding Eric Rakowski's approach to the just allocation of resources in mental health care.[1] Resource distribution, he argues, ideally should be governed by the independent and informed choices of individuals who need mental health services. In this view, many difficult moral dilemmas disappear as health care decisions are dictated by the wishes of patients who are free to make good decisions, to assume risks, or to make poor judgments regarding their health care and insurance coverage. Similarly, fewer problems will be encountered by health care systems, he argues, if they are designed to respect individual choice more fully and are not required to provide services for patients who, for example, have chosen no or minimal insurance. This emphasis on the principle of autonomy necessarily relies on a second principle of fairness—such as fair opportunities to obtain health insurance or fair opportunities to seek and pay for chosen treatments. Ultimately, suggests Rakowski, justice should serve to "restore as nearly as possible the fair footing"[2] of those who are unfortunate with those who have been luckier in life and illness. This approach is both thoughtful and compelling. Its limitations, however, appear in the everyday reality that mental health services often are needed by individuals whose autonomy may be compromised and for whom life and illness have been, and will continue to be, unfair.

In this chapter, we first outline how we understand Rakowski's proposal in relation to resource allocation for mental illness treatment in our society, and then we explain how the proposal is not attuned to the realities experienced by mentally ill individuals and the professionals who care for them.

Key Elements of the Proposal

Rakowski's basic idea is that resources should be distributed according to the informed choices of individuals who have a fair chance at health resources despite illness or social disadvantage. He argues that in a world such as ours, where *need for care exceeds resources for care*, "the only fair way to frame a policy for deciding [resource allocation] is by appealing to what was or what would have been the free choice of those who are subject to the policy".[3] Rakowski opposes intrusive governmental paternalism regarding individual health care choices. He suggests that "no one will be worse off, and some will be better off, if people have the liberty to decide for themselves,"[4] arguing against, for example, government-mandated, expensive, universal insurance policies. Favoring the principles of autonomy and fairness, Rakowski also cautions against the view that need alone entitles people to receive full health services. Severity of illness or degree of suffering, he suggests, should not be the values that drive the distribution of health care resources. Instead, the patient's preferences and prior planning (e.g., selection of an insurance package with more or less coverage, according to one's personal values) in a system of fair opportunities for choice should determine the health services he or she later receives.

As physical and mental problems are both species of bad luck, Rakowski suggests that they are not intrinsically different. In this way affirming the concerns of the mentally ill, Rakowski argues that "justice requires evening out the effects of people's undeserved good or ill fortune insofar as that is practicable".[5] Rakowski acknowledges, however, that disagreements exist about how to distribute resources to those who face greater health risks and suffering through no fault of their own (i.e., the "unlucky") or to those who are unable to make autonomous, informed, "competent" choices concerning their health care and insurance (such as children and some people with mental illness). He reports four possible responses: (1) improve the situation of disadvantaged individuals without causing undue hardship to others; (2) provide the level of health care and insurance coverage to "incompetent" individuals as would be selected by those who are "competent"; (3) provide resources that will relieve only the worst suffering of children and the most severely compromised mentally ill; and (4) do nothing to address the discrepancies between the fortunate and the unfortunate, including children and the mentally ill who are decisionally compromised. Though apparently favoring the first two more humane responses, Rakowski does not offer a simple solution. Instead he suggests that such issues must be considered in the context of a larger discussion governed by concepts such as the appropriateness of minimal governmental paternalism (e.g., vaccinations, basic mandatory insurance), the inappropriateness of more pervasive paternalism, and the unlucky individual's responsibilities toward others.

Rakowski then explores the ramifications of his approach in several areas. With respect to the highly debated problem of personal responsibility for illness, Rakowski argues that fault becomes a nonissue in his scheme. In a system where people can exercise choice in their insurance coverage, their later care and the health care resources they receive are dictated by their prior decisions: "It is their preferences as insurance buyers, not the morality of their actions that determine what care they receive."[6] Similarly, the dilemmas pertaining to how to allocate a very limited, desperately needed resource to competing individuals ("fair chances/best outcomes") or restricted resources to competing groups with differing levels of benefit (the "aggregation" problem) become straightforward: resource assignment, again, is determined by each patient's prior insurance choice.

In Rakowski's view, insurance choice represents an autonomous decision made by the patient that should be respected and implemented. Complications arise, he acknowledges, when choices are made badly or are based on poor information. Nevertheless, he asserts that medical resources limited principally because of human choice and not nature should be allocated through the exercise of autonomous choice and should not be "governed by principles that give weight to randomness, differential outcomes, and other factors."[7]

Rakowski's proposal in relation to mental health care falls into five areas: private mental health insurance, preexisting conditions, paying for care for the chronically mentally ill, public mental health insurance, and bipolar patients and the "aggregation" problem.

Private Mental Health Insurance

Here Rakowski comments that "in a just world, private insurance is best seen as an autonomy-respecting substitute for the more comprehensive insurance against misfortune that justice otherwise mandates."[8] He believes that restrictions on mental health coverage are not inherently unjust, and he questions whether in fact mental illness gets short shrift in private health insurance plans. Rakowski wonders how insurance plans can be crafted, given the variety of human choices and values with respect to mental illness. He argues that the government should not enforce private mental health insurance but raises the problem of how to handle the situation of patients who make poor coverage choices and then become desperately ill, "unfairly" placing the burden of care upon others.

Preexisting Conditions

Rakowski believes that "people who are set back through no fault of their own are entitled *at the very least* to insure against poor mental health on the same terms as everybody else" and that unlucky individuals who suffer "from a young age are entitled *at the very least* to whatever compensation would be provided by the insurance policies that most competent people buy for themselves."[9] He favors a tax incentive for unlucky individuals as a way to bring their situation closer to that of more fortunate individuals. He also supports setting similar insurance rates for both healthy individuals and those who have "preexisting conditions" as another method of creating greater fairness.

Paying for the Care of the Chronically Mentally Ill

Rakowski offers three responses to the question of who should pay for the care of the chronically ill: a) the sufferers themselves; b) the government, through taxes for all; and c) government-mandated private insurance. He then discards the first response, stating that it is not justifiable on practical and philosophical grounds to insist that all individuals buy health insurance. Instead, "in a world such as ours, marked by an unjust distribution of resources,"[10] Rakowski favors an approach that combines the second and third responses. He proposes a system requiring that people who have adequate resources select and purchase private insurance and that "at least some" people pay taxes to provide physical and mental health care to poor individuals.

Public Mental Health Insurance

Rakowski suggests that a mandatory, public mental health scheme is "consonant" with "virtually any rights-based theory of distributive justice paired with moderate paternalism, so long as the costs [are] properly apportioned."[11] Rakowski then raises many questions ranging from how much money should be set aside, who should pay, who should receive, how much should the recipients get, who should administer the programs, and the like. He argues that autonomy-based, informed-choice approaches eliminate many moral problems, because individuals decide for themselves about tough future decisions. He does not answer what he defines as "the only difficult moral judgment"—the question of whether to give special consideration to the unlucky, incompetent individuals (children and the mentally ill) who were not able to "protect themselves, either by acting responsibly or by insuring" before misfortune struck.[12]

Bipolar Patients and the Aggregation Problem

Here Rakowski states that multiple uncertainties besetting clinicians may be translated into the following single concrete question: "If a clinician must decide to help one bipolar patient, five unipolar depressed patients, or ten patients suffering from panic disorder, how should she spend her time?"[13] He offers no answer, deferring to clinical issues, but he then expresses concern over the inequities in the current system of mental health care in which short-term care occurs through "private arrangements" and long-term care through public programs: "One's objection must be to the underlying distribution of wealth and income," however, and not to the delegation of services to private and public sectors.[14] Finally, Rakowski repeats his basic concept that mental health care should be distributed by patients' "antecedent, informed preferences" not by independent moral principles, such as the injunction that we ought to help the worst off first.[15]

Rakowski's ultimate conclusion is poignant for clinicians: he acknowledges what he believes to be an understandable "longing" for a "clearer rule" that may simplify clinical judgments in relation to resource allocation. Offering what he describes as perhaps "meager" advice, he sees no way to lessen the clinician's "predicament." He states that "it is impossible to write rules to cover every treatment decision in advance."[16] The predicament of the mental health clinician within the larger health system's predicament will be discussed in the following sections.

Autonomy and Fairness in Caring for People with Mental Illness

We all have sufficient strength to endure the misfortunes of others.
—Francis, Duc de La Rochefoucauld

Prediction is very difficult, especially about the future.
—Niels Bohr

Mental illnesses are not a neat, fair, and orderly set of diseases affecting autonomous adults. Mental illnesses affect young adults before they have had the opportunity to accumulate the wisdom and wealth necessary to select "appropriate" insurance. Many mental illnesses affect children. The parents of some of these children are mentally ill with few resources and may also have serious symptoms affecting their judgment. Mental illness often coincides with underlying developmental disabilities, physical health problems, and addictions, creating extraordinary challenges for self-care and self-advocacy. The experience of being mentally ill affects one's insight, character development, and expressions of self in the world. Mental illness, by definition, affects the whole of one's life, leading to deterioration in one's social and societal roles; it is not a tightly contained problem that can be excised like a tumor or eradicated with chemotherapy.

Mental health clinicians respond to these realities each day and consequently will see Rakowski's views in relation to mental illness as naïve at best, ill-informed at worst. Although his proposal thoughtfully addresses resource allocation issues for the majority of individuals who experience good health and routine medical conditions—individuals for whom autonomous decision making and fair opportunities may be possible—the limitations of the approach he offers become most salient when one considers the enormity and true nature of clinical care involving the many individuals who suffer from mental illness. This represents 50 million adults in the United States alone, of which approximately half receive mental health services.[17] Moreover, it has been estimated that nearly half of all individuals will develop a significant mental disorder such as major depression, schizophrenia and other psychotic illnesses, alcohol or drug dependence, or generalized anxiety disorder during their lifetime. The most severe of these illnesses, by their very nature, may cause cognitive deficits, diminish insight, compromise judgment, erode personal autonomy, misguide life choices, interfere with decisional abilities, disrupt communication, and alter other fundamental expressions of the self.[18] Seriously mentally ill people are more likely than other ill individuals to exist along the margins of society, where issues of fairness and autonomy pale in relation to the matters of everyday survival and where only institutionalization offers occasional respite.[19] Those who are less profoundly ill also struggle greatly—living less productive, less empowered, less pleasurable, and fundamentally more limited lives. In this context, freedom of choice and fairness of opportunity are arguably diminished in comparison with those who are not ill or otherwise vulnerable. These are the individuals tentatively approached along the edges of Rakowski's proposal but are central to the special task of mental health care.

Examination of informed consent in clinical care illustrates several of the problems in the proposal offered by Rakowski. Informed consent is salient because this practice standard represents the principal safeguard for patient autonomy in our system of health care. Informed consent is the process by which patients and care providers together approach diagnostic and therapeutic decision making. Fulfillment of informed consent in clinical practice is a complex, iterative task. It is not merely a signature on a form or a single conversation in isolation from other aspects of the therapeutic relationship. Ideally, consent occurs within the context of an alliance between the caregiver and patient that is characterized by trust, truthfulness, and faithfulness to serving the best interests and well-being of the patient.[20]

The consent process itself is constituted by several elements, as depicted in figure 6.1. First is *disclosure of information* by the physician regarding the nature of the patient's illness, the alternatives for evaluation and treatment, and the risks, benefits, and expected outcomes of possible treatments and, importantly, of nontreatment at the time. Second is the *patient's genuine understanding* of this information and *appreciation* of its personal meaning, given the circumstances of his or her life. This involves the ability to communicate preferences, to understand and logically work with the facts of the illness and the intervention. It also involves the ability to discern the meaning of the decision and its implications. Taken together, these abilities comprise *intact decisional ability* with respect to health care decisions. Finally, informed consent hinges upon the expression of the authentic, uncoerced choice of the ill individual, or *true voluntariness*.[21] This ambitious task is best understood as a process within the patient-clinician relationship in which clinical issues and personal values are clarified.

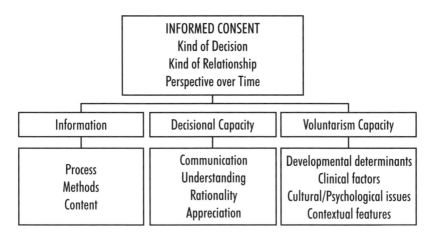

FIGURE 6.1   ELEMENTS OF INFORMED CONSENT

Source: Adapted from L. W. Roberts, "Ethics and Mental Illness Research," in *Psychiatric Clinics of North America* 25, no. 3 (2002):525–45.

Far from this ideal, empirical studies of informed consent suggest that it is a goal that is seldom fully attained. More than 400 studies have been performed over three decades to explore the practice of consent in clinical and research contexts, and it has been well demonstrated that barriers to optimal consent practices exist.[22] An early study by Cassileth and colleagues, for example, found that only 60 percent of 200 cancer patients who had agreed to a significant procedure (chemotherapy, radiation therapy, or surgery) recalled the purpose and nature of the procedure one day after informed consent was obtained. Fewer patients, 55 percent, could identify accurately even one of the possible major risks of the procedure.[23] Other studies reviewed by Meisel and Roth indicate that practical issues such as physician and patient attitudes, communication problems, incomplete disclosure of information, poor recall by patients, complex medical language, rushed or inappropriate timing, inaccurate assumptions, impaired decisional abilities, and patient vulnerabilities may conspire to undermine the consent process.[24] When the issue of informed consent by proxy decision makers is examined, significant discrepancies exist between patients' personal choices and their proxies' choices for them. These studies, taken together, illuminate how the concept of autonomy in decision making—even when conscientiously undertaken—is not easily translated to medical and psychiatric clinical practice.[25]

In comparing the abilities of physically versus mentally ill individuals with respect to consent decisions, as expected, the mentally ill individuals appear to have greater difficulty. These deficits may at times be temporized by treatment or by improved consent procedures, but the problems of informed consent are amplified for psychiatric patients for three reasons. First, their illnesses may lead to fluctuations or deterioration in cognitive abilities, insight, judgment, and communication skills. Second, mental illnesses can give rise to feelings of desperation not unlike those experienced by people with terminal illnesses or chronic and severe physical pain. This level of dire need creates special vulnerabilities and results in tremendous dependence on health care providers and institutions. This situation inherently leads to diminished voluntariness and in some cases may invite exploitation. Third, the doctor-patient relationship often differs in the care of the severely mentally ill and entails exceptional respectfulness and scrupulousness on the part of the clinician. In particular, sound clinical care of patients with psychiatric illnesses at times requires that physicians exert power in ways that usurp patient autonomy to protect and treat their patients properly.[26] Moreover, psychiatrically ill patients may at times pose greater burdens and dangers to their families and to society at large than do medically ill patients, which places greater responsibilities on physicians to intervene. Consequently, special efforts to utilize power ethically—such as peer review and specialist consultation with difficult patients or judicial procedures related to involuntary hospitalization, determinations of "competence," and appointment of treatment guardians—have been developed and are intrinsic to the standard of psychiatric care practiced throughout the United States.[27] These three issues make the task of obtaining informed consent particularly meaningful and challenging in the care of the mentally ill, a reality not accommodated by Rakowski's proposal.

Other empirical work suggests the fallibility of adopting an idealized view of the autonomous decisions of individuals.[28] For example, some evidence suggests that people make different decisions in real life as opposed to hypothetical situations. This, we suggest, is analogous to prospective insurance selection. The discrepancy between what people can envision as necessary and what people actually need in a time of suffering renders Rakowski's schema as ecologically invalid, as a theory without grounding in real life. In contrast with theoreticians, clinicians will naturally place greater emphasis on their understanding of the intrinsic vulnerabilities of patienthood when designing a system. Clinicians will recognize that personal autonomy around health care is iterative; it emerges through multiple interactions and does not manifest itself in a single event such as the moment of insurance selection, as Rakowski's proposal implies. Indeed, the single decision of insurance choice is one beginning, not the end, of autonomous decision making in health care.

Beyond the matter of autonomy, fairness is also elusive in mental health care. Becoming ill, experiencing pain, and suffering are intrinsically experienced as unfair by all patients. Because of the loss of self and the tremendous stigma accompanying many psychiatric diseases, this unfairness is amplified in the daily interactions of the mentally ill person.[29] Second, it has been documented that treatments for psychiatric illnesses are *more* or are *equally* effective when compared to available treatments for certain medical illnesses, specifically angioplasty and antihypertensive therapies. Valuable biological and psychosocial interventions have been developed for schizophrenia, bipolar disorder, major depression, panic disorder, and disorders affecting children and the elderly.[30] In light of these data, it is ironic—and fundamentally inequitable—that there is less public acceptance and greater reluctance around reimbursement for psychiatric treatments. Third, part of how psychiatric diagnoses are understood relates to their impact on patients' abilities to function.[31] Deterioration in ordinary coping at work and in personal relationships is essential to the definition of mental illness. Schizophrenia patients who derive originally from all sorts of socioeconomic backgrounds (1 percent of all people in the world), for example, experience decline so severe that they are eventually overrepresented among the homeless and the poor. Consequently, they "unfairly" lack both resources and opportunities to improve their situation. Throughout his proposal, Rakowski predicates much on its implementation "in a just world." He clearly understands that this is an idealized view but may not fully appreciate just how very *unjust* the world is for the mentally ill.

This discussion serves to demonstrate how reasonable and thoughtful ideas applicable to the physically ill or perhaps the most mildly mentally ill are not appropriate in the care of most mentally ill individuals. Consequently, special differences in the nature of mental health care must be accommodated by both the structure of services and the resource allocation strategies implemented.[32] Moreover, clinicians must have a clear and valued voice in the design of these services and strategies if they are to be attuned and effective.[33]

Conclusion

Rakowski presents a compelling and valuable proposal for a scheme of just health care resource allocation that emphasizes autonomy and fairness. Its greatest strengths are the respect it accords individuals and the importance it places upon equity. Rakowski envisions a system in which people have opportunities, are free to make choices, and then must live with them. Clinical experience with mentally ill patients demands a more measured view of autonomy and fairness. We suggest that transitioning to a new, just resource allocation strategy entails a coherent, organized, collaborative effort involving individuals and institutions with shared, compatible interests. Understanding access issues and the unique concerns surrounding human suffering are crucial, as are concerns about equity for those patients to be served optimally by the system. There must be adequate insight about the roles, responsibilities, autonomy, and accountability of the different participants of the system, including physicians and patients. Most importantly, its design must be clinically astute and forward-looking and must dedicate itself to prevention, education, and research in order to be enduring and successful. For these reasons, we regretfully conclude that Rakowski's approach neglects attunement to clinical realities. His theoretical approach omits some fundamental issues that are crucial to the successful development of a new, just, and enduring system that is humane, clinically and scientifically sound, and beneficial to mentally ill patients despite limited resources.

Informed consent is influenced by the nature of the decision (e.g., clinical or research, acute or nonacute), the kind of relationship in which the consent process occurs, and changing perspectives toward the choice over time.

Information

Accurate and balanced information regarding several issues is communicated in an informed consent process, such as the anticipated risks and benefits of the intervention (or treatment), alternatives and their expected outcomes (including no intervention at all), who is responsible for various steps, and possible interventions in case of serious side effects or complications. Consent communication ordinarily occurs as an ongoing process, and it may be enhanced by various methods (e.g., multiple conversations, written educational materials, or videos).

Decisional Capacity

The requirements for decisional capacity are that the individual be able to express a preference (i.e., capacity for expression or communication), to take in and understand relevant information (i.e., capacity for comprehension), to think through the choice at hand in a way that is "rational" and deliberate (i.e., capacity for reasoning or rational thinking), and, most importantly, to make sense of the decision and its consequences within the context of the individual's personal history, values, emotions, and context (i.e., capacity for appreciation).

Voluntarism

Voluntarism encompasses the individual's ability to act in accord with one's authentic sense of what is good, right, and best in light of one's situation, values, and prior history. Deliberateness, purposefulness of intent, clarity, genuineness, and coherence with prior life decisions are implicitly emphasized in this construction. We have proposed that the capacity for voluntarism may be assessed according to four dimensions: (a) developmental determinants, (b) clinical factors, (c) cultural/psychological issues, and (d) contextual features.

Notes

1. See Eric Rakowski, "The Just Allocation of Mental Health Care," chapter 4 in this book.

2. Ibid.
3. Ibid.
4. Ibid.
5. Ibid.
6. Ibid.
7. Ibid.
8. Ibid.
9. Ibid.
10. Ibid.
11. Ibid.
12. Ibid.
13. Ibid.
14. Ibid.
15. Ibid.
16. Ibid.
17. U.S. Department of Health and Human Services, *Mental Health: A Report of the Surgeon General—Executive Summary* (Rockville, Md.: U.S. Department of Health and Human Services, Substance Abuse and Mental Health Services Administration, Center for Mental Health Services, National Institutes of Health, National Institute of Mental Health, 1999).
18. D. A. Regier et al., "The De Facto U.S. Mental and Addictive Disorders Service System. Epidemiologic Catchment Area Prospective 1-Year Prevalence Rates of Disorders and Services," *Archives of General Psychiatry* 50, no. 2 (1993): 85–94; F. Redlich and S. R. Kellert, "Trends in American Mental Health," in *Issues in Health Services*, ed. S. J. Williams (New York: Wiley, 1980), 121–31; L. W. Roberts, "Ethics and Mental Illness Research," *Psychiatric Clinics of North America* 25, no. 3 (2002): 525–45.
19. F. Arnoff, "Social Consequences of Policy toward Mental Illness," *Science* 188 (1975): 1277–81; L. W. Roberts et al., "Persons with Mental Illness," in *Managed Care*, ed. D. A. Bennahum (Cleveland, Ohio: Pilgrim Press, 1999), 184–208.
20. L. W. Roberts, "Informed Consent and Care," in *International Encyclopedia of the Social and Behavioral Sciences*, ed. N. J. Smelser and P. B. Baltes (Oxford, England: Elsevier Science, Ltd., 2002), 12296–302.
21. L. W. Roberts, "Informed Consent and the Capacity for Voluntarism," *American Journal of Psychiatry* 159, no. 5 (2002): 705–12.
22. J. Sugarman et al., "Empirical Research on Informed Consent. An Annotated Bibliography," *Hastings Center Report* 29, no. 1 (January–February 1999): S1–42; C. Lidz et al., "Barriers to Informed Consent," *Annals of Internal Medicine* 99, no. 4 (1983): 539–43.
23. B. Cassileth et al., "Informed Consent—Why Are Its Goals Imperfectly Realized?" *New England Journal of Medicine* 302 (1980): 896–900.
24. A. Meisel and L. H. Roth, "What We Do and Do Not Know about Informed Consent," *Journal of the American Medical Association* 246, no. 21 (1981): 2473–77.

25. Sugarman et al., "Empirical Research on Informed Consent"; J. W. Warren et al., "Informed Consent by Proxy: An Issue in Research with Elderly Patients," *New England Journal of Medicine* 315, no. 18 (1986): 1124–28; G. A. Sachs et al., "Ethical Aspects of Dementia Research: Informed Consent and Proxy Consent," *Clinical Research* 42, no. 3 (1994): 403–12.

26. L. Roberts and B. Roberts, "Psychiatric Research Ethics: An Overview of Evolving Guidelines and Current Ethical Dilemmas in the Study of Mental Illness," *Biological Psychiatry* 46, no. 8 (1999): 1025–38.

27. M. Angell, "Respecting the Autonomy of Competent Patients," *New England Journal of Medicine* 310, no. 17 (1984): 1115–16.

28. Sugerman et al., "Empirical Research on Informal Consent."

29. U.S. Department of Health and Human Services, *Mental Health*; Roberts et al., "Persons with Mental Illness"; S. K. Severino and H. Chung, "Health Care Reform: Implications for Academic Psychiatric Institutions," *Journal of Mental Health Administration* 22, no. 1 (1995): 77–84.

30. S. Keith and S. Matthews, "The Value of Psychiatric Treatment: Its Efficacy in Severe Mental Disorders," *Psychopharmacology Bulletin* 29, no. 4 (1993): 427–30.

31. Sugerman et al., "Empirical Research on Informal Consent."

32. Severino and Chung, "Health Care Reform"; J. E. Sabin, "A Credo for Ethical Managed Care in Mental Health Practice," *Hospital and Community Psychiatry* 45, no. 9 (1994): 859–60.

33. M. Siegler, "Decision-Making Strategy for Clinical-Ethical Problems in Medicine," *Archives of Internal Medicine* 142, no. 12 (1982): 2178–79.

CHAPTER 7

The Democracy Problem in Mental Health Care Priority Setting

Dan W. Brock

THROUGHOUT THE WORLD countries are facing more explicitly the problem of scarcity in health care. As the growth of health care costs continues to outstrip the growth in national or personal income and in the rate of inflation, health care absorbs an ever-increasing proportion of national and personal income. Because nearly all developed countries have some form of national health care or universal health insurance, the worldwide debates about how to control the growth of health care spending inevitably become political debates about spending in public programs. In the United States the health care system is much more heterogeneous, including public health insurance programs such as Medicare and Medicaid, fee-for-service private insurance plans, as well as a variety of capitation and managed care plans, together with 41 million Americans without any form of health insurance. This diversity has made the debate in the United States about controlling the growth of health care costs more complex, envisaging cost control taking place in very different financing and delivery settings. Despite these differences in the context in which cost control debates take place, both in the United States and around the world, one common denominator is the increasingly explicit recognition that it is no longer possible or reasonable to deny that resources for health care are scarce or to insist that we should provide all beneficial care to everyone, no matter how small the benefit and how great the cost. Priorities must be set, and in this sense health care must be rationed.

In the United States, the public and professionals alike are going through a fundamental change in their expectations, entitlements, and responsibilities regarding the health care that can or should be made available to patients, a process of change where duration will be measured in years or even decades. The debate over these changes is likely to be more intense in the United States than in many other countries for various reasons, among them because we have traditionally employed a fee-for-service system of organization and financing of health care containing economic, professional, and even moral incentives that encouraged both physicians and patients to ignore the scarcity of resources.

Explicit priority-setting processes are one means of confronting this scarcity and of making decisions about how to accommodate to it.

In an influential article a decade ago, Norman Daniels distinguished several substantive distributive issues that arise when we attempt to set priorities in health care: the conflict between best outcomes and fair chances; what priority, if any, to give to the needs of the worst off; and the aggregation problem—when should small benefits to many persons have priority over large benefits to fewer persons.[1] Daniels quite correctly notes both that most traditional general principles or theories of distributive justice are too indeterminate to provide full solutions to these problems and that we lack a theory of rationing that would provide bridge principles between problems of institutional design and more general principles of justice. I believe the difficulty is, if anything, worse than this. Work by moral philosophers on these moral issues, as well as on other rationing problems that Daniels did not discuss,[2] is at a very early stage of development.[3] Not only do we lack solutions to Daniels's problems that have gained any wide consensus, but we have not yet even clarified the range of reasonable positions on the problems and the nature of the moral considerations that divide those positions. And yet any prioritization process or allocational principles for health care resources inevitably must take positions on them, whether they do so explicitly or only implicitly. It is our lack of adequate principles and agreed-on solutions to these problems that gives rise to at least part of the fourth problem Daniels identified, which he called the democracy problem.

The Democracy Problem

Daniels's characterization of the democracy problem suggests that it is not in fact a single question but several related questions: (1) In the absence of any principled solutions to these rationing problems, to what extent can we rely on fair democratic procedures as the only way to determine what constitutes a fair rationing outcome? (2) What would be fair democratic procedures for use on these problems? (3) To what extent is reliance on a democratic process to resolve these problems a matter of pure procedural justice or instead impure or imperfect procedural justice? (4) If the latter, when there is a conflict between the outcomes of fair procedures and people's moral convictions about particular cases or their general moral principles, how much weight should we give to each?[4]

These questions raise extremely difficult and complex issues in moral and political philosophy to which I have nothing even approaching complete answers or positions, but in this article I will at least begin to explore them, mostly in their more general form concerning health care generally, but with some eye to their specific shape in mental health care prioritization. However, a few points or qualifications need to be made before we address these questions directly. First, it is a mistake to think that a single account of what would be fair democratic procedures is possible. Fair democratic procedures might simply be general democratic political procedures, such as a legislature's employing majority rule voting procedures. If prioritization procedures with some claim to a democratic pedigree are located within the health care system, they might, nevertheless, be part of very different health care systems or exist at different places within some particular health care system. For example, in a national health care system such as that in the ill-fated Clinton proposal, a National Health Board, appointed by the president but responsive to the political process, was to make determinations of medical necessity concerning treatments for particular conditions.[5] In the Oregon Medicaid prioritization process, ordinary citizens were polled to determine the weights to be assigned to different functional or disability states in its adaptation of the Quality of Well-Being Scale.[6] In a managed care plan, a committee made up of the various stakeholders could be employed to develop practice guidelines and standards for treatments to be covered or provided by the plan. Note that the complexity here comes both from the different institutional contexts in which Daniels's rationing problems arise and from the quite different questions or issues that comprise those problems. In a highly heterogeneous health care system such as that in the United States, there can be no single answer to question 2 mentioned earlier about what would constitute fair democratic procedures. I believe that the most we can hope for is to identify either some features of different procedures that would make them fair and democratic or different interests people have in the political procedures that address rationing problems.

A second preliminary point concerns the idea of fair democratic procedures in the question at issue here. In everyday experience and in political philosophy, "democracy" is what has been called a "contested concept"—what counts as democracy is controversial, but because democracy is a widely favored form of government, proponents of many different forms of government have been eager to capture the label of democracy for their favorite form. A widely accepted component of democracy is the participation of citizens, either directly or through representatives, in making political decisions by a majority rule procedure. But if democracy is understood as purely procedurally in this way, as referring to some form of majoritarian decision procedure used by citizens or their representatives, then it should be clear that our own political traditions in the United States reject this pure democracy. We have procedural limits on majorities working their will; for example, procedural rules in the Senate, such as the closure rules on debate that give filibustering minorities the power to block majorities' actions and the veto power of the president that can only be overridden by two-thirds majorities in both the House and the Senate. We also have strong substantive limits on majorities effectuating their will. The Bill of Rights and such provisions as the equal protection clause of the 14th Amend-

ment to the Constitution provide grounds for the courts to strike down legislation passed by majorities that violates these constitutionally protected fundamental rights. In international contexts, the emphasis on human rights also
constitutes a rejection of democracy in this pure procedural form.

These general procedural and substantive limits on majoritarian decision procedures constitute a rejection of pure democracy in our moral and political traditions in order to protect fundamental rights against unjust infringement by
majorities. A comparable constraint on procedures for making just or fair health
care rationing decisions would be a right to health care that democratic majorities would not be permitted to infringe. But if democratic procedures for making
rationing decisions require, to be fair or just, an independent and prior account
of the right to health care, then they presuppose at least part of what they were
to be used to produce. An uncontroversial substantive account of the right to
health care that is sufficiently detailed to solve the rationing problems is exactly
what we lack, and it is what we turn to fair democratic procedures to determine.
We cannot settle the matter of what are fair democratic procedures until we
have substantive principles defining a right to health care, the lack of which the
appeal to democratic procedures was designed to remedy. We shall return to this
difficulty.

The last general preliminary point is the worry that appeal to real-world
democratic procedures to set priorities, instead of moral principles and objective
measures of burdens of disease, risks giving weight to ignorance, prejudices, and
discrimination that infect democratic decision processes. This is a particular
worry in mental health care, where many forms of mental illness remain the subject of strong and common prejudices and often seriously stigmatize those who
have them. If someone directly displayed these prejudices, for example, by saying that we need not be concerned about the health care needs of "crazies" and
"junkies," we would regard this as prejudice that should not influence health care
priorities. But as Ronald Dworkin has argued in a different context, it is often
difficult even in theory, and certainly in practice, to separate people's legitimate
preferences and values concerning mental illness and disability from prejudices
and false beliefs about them and the people who have them.[7] Any procedural
solution to setting priorities for mental health care must keep these prejudices
and false beliefs from infecting the procedures and, in turn, the results. With
these preliminary points noted, I turn more directly to the democracy problem.

Is the Democracy Problem a Problem of Error?

Daniels first characterizes the democracy problem as a problem of error:

> A fair democratic process, or a methodology that rests on the expression
> of preferences, leads to judgments that deviate from either intuitive or

theoretically based judgments about the relative importance of certain health outcomes or services. The problem is how much weight to give the intuitive or theoretically based judgments as opposed to the expressed preferences.[8]

But it is misleading, if not mistaken, to characterize this as a problem of decisions that deviate from the truth. That presupposes exactly what we do not have and what drives us to appeal to democratic procedures or the expression of preferences—an agreed-upon standard by which errors can be identified and measured. For example, Oregon used telephone surveys to obtain ordinary citizens' judgments about the relative reduction in well-being or quality of life from a variety of disease conditions or disabilities. Implicit in that process was the assumption that either there is no objectively correct standard that determines the relative level of well-being for different functional limitations or at least no evaluations of those limitations widely accepted as objectively correct; Oregon appealed instead to the evaluations of a (purportedly) average group of Oregon citizens. (This is not to say that there were not some apparent internal inconsistencies or anomalous results in Oregon's ranking, such as those Daniels cites.) For such evaluations then, it is misleading to characterize the democracy problem as a problem of error because there was no standard by which to establish them as in error. That was at least one reason why a democratic process of soliciting the value judgments of a group of representative citizens was employed.

One might argue that it was for reasons of democratic theory that Oregon appealed to the value judgments of its citizens, not because there are no standards for determining when those value judgments are correct. Democratic legitimacy, not value indeterminacy, required that consultative process. But in the case of clearly empirical or factual data necessary to the process, such as the average cost of providing a particular treatment to a patient in a particular condition or how many such patients were treated in the most recent year in Oregon's Medicaid program, no one considered relying on the beliefs of a representative group of Oregon citizens. Those beliefs would in virtually all cases have been formed without the relevant data and so would have been mistaken; instead, Oregon gathered the available data from experts so as to minimize the possibility of using mistaken estimates of the cost or frequency of different treatments. When the questions are agreed to be uncontroversial empirical or factual matters, few dispute that uninformed judgments should be corrected by relevant data and that it is important to devise procedures that will generally do so.

This is not to deny, of course, that relevant data often may be incomplete, imperfect, and controversial. But then the debate should be, and often is, about what the relevant data do or do not show, not whether we should instead rely on uninformed or mistaken beliefs in conflict with the data. Nor is this to deny that it is often difficult and controversial, in principle much less in practice, to determine whether a particular question concerns an empirical matter of fact or a personal or moral evaluation; when Oregon asked citizens to evaluate the relative quality of life with a particular disability, it would have been difficult in practice to distinguish in the individuals polled their factual beliefs about the effects on one's life of having a particular disability from their evaluations of the relative importance of those effects or of the overall quality of the resulting life. Nor finally is it to deny that particular individuals will not sometimes believe that others are mistaken in their value and moral judgments—for example, either about the relative quality of life with a particular disability or about issues such as how much priority, if any, should be given to the worst off in allocating health care resources. From a standpoint within a particular moral conception, other conflicting moral positions will often be seen as mistaken. But it is to say that for at least many such judgments, there are no generally accepted evaluative or moral standards by which individual citizens' judgments, or the outcomes of democratic procedures, could be agreed to be mistaken and so properly corrected or set aside. Moral issues such as Daniels's first three rationing problems are likely to remain, at least to a significant degree, contested and controversial; they are examples in the domain of justice and rationing of the permanent "fact of pluralism" at the heart of liberal political theory.

I should not be understood as claiming that all value or moral questions are so irretrievably contested that democracies properly settle them all procedurally, for example, by majority vote. That is not my view, and it is certainly not our democratic political tradition, as I have already noted; fundamental rights such as those in the Bill of Rights properly constrain democratic majorities in the actions they can take. But at least now, and I believe for the foreseeable future, detailed solutions to Daniels's first three rationing problems will remain seriously controversial. We will lack any widely accepted standard, in either people's "intuitive or theoretically based judgments" by which the preferences or judgments of others or the outcomes of democratic procedures could justifiably be corrected or set aside as mistaken. The proper role for individuals' intuitions or theoretically based judgments is in public and political deliberation and debate within fair democratic procedures about the moral problems posed by rationing. Thus, the democracy problem in its most fundamental form is not a problem of error, as the fourth of the related questions by which Daniels characterizes it would suggest, and we must look to a different understanding of it.

Pure, Perfect, and Imperfect Procedural Justice

What kind of procedural justice is the use of a democratic process to resolve substantive rationing problems—pure procedural justice, perfect procedural justice, or imperfect procedural justice—and how does this affect the justification of appealing to procedures to resolve the rationing problems? First, what is the difference between these three forms of procedural justice? I shall follow John Rawls's statement of them.[9] A distribution is a matter of pure procedural justice if it has two properties: (1) we have no independent nonprocedural standard for what would be a just or fair distribution; (2) there is a procedure such that when it is followed, whatever distribution or outcome it produces will be fair. Rawls used the example of a fair gamble—if the terms and conditions of a gamble are fair—for example, the dice are not loaded or the cards are not marked— then if the procedures of the gamble are carried out, whatever distribution results will be fair. Distributions can fail to be a matter of pure procedural justice because either condition 1, 2, or both, is not satisfied. A distribution is a matter of perfect procedural justice if we have a substantive, nonprocedural standard for a fair outcome and also a procedure that is guaranteed to produce that outcome. A simple example is the division of a piece of cake between two children, neither of whom has any differential claims to it; the fair outcome is an equal division and the traditional procedure that should guarantee that result is letting one cut the cake and the other choose the first piece. A distribution is a matter of imperfect procedural justice if we have a substantive standard for a just or fair outcome, but there is no procedure that guarantees we will always reach that outcome. An example of distributing unwanted "bads" instead of desired "goods" is the criminal justice system. The standard is to impose punishment on all and only the guilty, but we know that there is no feasible procedure for determining who will be punished that will always reach that outcome; any feasible procedure will sometimes unintentionally punish the innocent or let the guilty go free or, more likely, both.

Before turning to what kind of procedural justice health care rationing choices are, we also need to distinguish whether a substantive, nonprocedural distributive standard is contested or uncontested. For example, the substantive distributive principle for the criminal justice system that all and only the guilty should be punished is widely uncontested and accepted; by contrast, given that the ideal standard cannot be met in practice, how to balance the risk of letting the guilty go free against the risk of punishing the innocent is highly contested.

How do these distinctions apply to the use of fair democratic procedures to settle the problems of health care rationing? And let us have before us at least one example of those problems—the priority to be given, if any, to the worst off or sickest at the cost of lower aggregate health benefits in prioritizing mental health care.[10] An example is the treatment of patients with severe, chronic schizophrenia versus patients with mild obsessive-compulsive disorder (OCD); the former are more seriously ill and worse off, but greater overall benefits might be produced by giving priority to the latter. The appeal to procedures is most defensible for questions of pure procedural justice; indeed, the appeal to procedures in these cases is indispensable because no alternative appeal to nonprocedural standards of justice is possible, and if the appropriate procedure is correctly followed no basis will exist for an objection that the outcome is unfair or unjust. However, none of Daniels's rationing problems, nor others that he does not discuss, are fully cases of pure procedural justice; for example, there are data that suggest most but not all people would give some priority to treating the sickest, which implies sometimes giving priority to treating severe schizophrenia over mild OCD.[11] But even people who are unsure to whom priority should be given do not believe there is a procedure that, if followed, would guarantee the fairness of its outcomes. In the case of a fair gamble, the point is not that we are unsure who should be the winner but instead that the winner should be whoever is designated as such when the procedure of the fair gamble is carried out. No one believes that the problems of health care rationing are like this—that there are no substantive outcome standards for the rationing problems, but that there is a procedure that if followed would guarantee that whatever results it produces are fair or just. Many people hold at least partial standards for fair resolutions of Daniels's rationing problems, although those standards are in most cases contested. This is most easily seen for utilitarians or consequentialists who believe that resources should always be allocated so as to maximize overall benefits to their beneficiaries; many health policy analysts and ordinary citizens believe that in the face of limited resources, we should use them in the manner that will produce the most good. This standard applies to each of Daniels's three rationing problems—it always permits aggregation of small benefits to many persons, gives no priority to the worst off, and always favors best outcomes over fair chances. Yet the utilitarian standard is notoriously controversial precisely in cases such as these.

Most problems of rationing and priority setting are also not cases of perfect but imperfect procedural justice. For example, consider Oregon's prioritization effort in its recent revision of its state Medicaid program.[12] To make the point succinctly, simplify their process by assuming that the final ranking of treatment-condition pairs was in terms of the relative benefits for the patients' well-being of each pair, as measured by the Oregon Health Services Commission's adaptation of Kaplan's Quality of Well-Being scale. (Complexities in the actual process, such as the "by hand" adjustments that commissioners made in the list produced by the data, probably made the procedure more imperfect.) Clearly this measure only imperfectly captures actual differences in patients' well-being. To give just one example, as critics of Oregon's efforts argued, treatment-condition pairs inevitably lump together cases in which there are significantly different effects on well-being from the same treatment due to sometimes subtle and complex differences between actual patients within each category.

Finally, and unfortunately for the appeal to procedures, all of Daniels's rationing problems are also cases in which the standards that real individuals apply to them to the extent that individuals have standards for them are often highly contested, reflecting deeper differences in moral theory and theories of distributive justice. People's moral judgments about particular cases of health care rationing, as well as the general principles they apply to such cases, are contested.

This means that we should be deeply skeptical that appeal to democratic procedures will produce just solutions to the problems of rationing. Those problems are not instances of pure procedural justice for which the appeal to procedures is uniquely suited. Moreover, even assuming uncontested standards for such problems, they are not problems of perfect procedural justice in which there is a procedure whose outcomes are guaranteed to meet those standards. Moreover, at least over a broad range of rationing problems, the standards for them are strongly contested; this means that there will often be no widely accepted basis for evaluating how imperfect specific decision procedures are, either on any particular occasion or in general. The appeal to procedures may be a practical compromise that most people will accept for priorities that need to be set and settled in real time; democratic procedures may be more likely to produce outcomes that will be generally accepted as reasonable compromises, but claims that such procedures can either determine what outcomes are just or produce just outcomes as measured against a generally accepted nonprocedural standard look to be unsupportable.

Three Places for the Appeal to Procedures

Nevertheless, even if rationing problems at best are largely issues of imperfect procedural justice on which the appeal to fair procedures is most problematic, there are three kinds of cases in which we might resort to fair procedures. First, there may be areas of indeterminacy in people's moral views where their moral principles either do not apply or where conflicting moral principles apply, but the relative weighting those principles should have is indeterminate over some range of cases (which I will call trade-off indeterminacy). Many people suffer trade-off indeterminacy in both the "fair chances versus best outcomes" problem and the "priority to the worst off versus best outcomes" problem; some, but indeterminate, weight must be given to each of the two conflicting considerations (although even that is controversial—utilitarians will give weight only to best outcomes). This fits Daniels's understanding of at least a part of the democracy problem as arising because principles or theories of distributive justice are too general to impose determinate solutions to the rationing problems. And it is hard to see how to make a principled defense of particular trade-offs between conflicting moral principles or values in the rationing problems that would be nonarbitrary and acceptable to most persons. There may turn out to be a significant range of overlapping indeterminacy over many rationing trade-offs in many or most people's moral views; for example, although for some cases many people will give more weight to best outcomes and others to fair chances, there may be other cases about which both groups are uncertain how to balance these conflicting moral considerations. These cases of common trade-off indeterminacy are a promising area for appeal to fair democratic procedures, although once again the boundaries of any such area will be controversial.

This picture of individuals' moral views containing a clearly demarcated range of cases in which they make specific determinate trade-offs, and likewise another clearly demarcated range of cases in which they are completely uncertain how to make trade-offs between the values or principles in conflict in rationing choices, is mistaken or is at least misleading. What is missing is the great variability in the degree of confidence individuals have in judgments about how to trade off these conflicting principles or values in different cases. Other things being equal, the less confidence an individual has in a particular rationing trade-off, the stronger the case for acknowledging that it is a trade-off about which reasonable people can disagree. Rationing cases or trade-offs about which it is acknowledged that reasonable people can disagree is a second promising area in which we might appeal to fair democratic procedures to resolve those disagreements, although once again which cases engender reasonable disagreement will be controversial.

There is a third, more problematic kind of case in which we often resort to democratic procedures to resolve deep and sharp moral and political differences between people and between groups. These are cases in which the conflicting parties often do not consider the issue, one about which reasonable people can disagree, but instead consider an issue in which some parties are correct and others are mistaken. Profound and often deeply divisive questions such as whether to declare war, to preserve wilderness areas, to do research on embryos, or to permit euthanasia are all left ultimately to the democratic political process to resolve. We might then also leave equally profound and divisive rationing disagreements to democratic political processes for resolution.

How should we think of the outcomes of the use of fair democratic procedures to resolve rationing problems in cases of overlapping indeterminacy, reasonable disagreement, or deeply divisive disagreement? Common to the three kinds of cases is lack of agreement about the proper trade-offs between conflicting moral claims, values, or principles. When issues of justice are at stake, we need a means of arriving at public policy which is fair or just to all affected by it, despite the lack of consensus on the substantive standards by which the fairness or justice of the policy can be assessed. The natural suggestion is that fair procedures could be a means of arriving at a fair compromise that all could accept.

What Are Fair Procedures for Rationing Decisions?

The moral case for resorting to procedural solutions of rationing problems depends, of course, on the moral quality of the procedures employed. If we resort only to the push and pull of and the deal making between different interest groups and political forces, then there would be no reason to assume that the outcome of this process has any moral claim to provide a fair or just resolution of rationing problems. If it is only a contest in which the most powerful political interests win the day, then that provides no moral support of the result. General acceptance of the political outcome may be preferable to continued social conflict and irresolution of the issues, but that changes the subject from just rationing to political accommodation. We need a process for rationing problems in which the issues of justice are addressed in a manner that morally supports accepting as just the outcomes of that process. We can use the literature of democratic theory to help make clear what is needed.

In the literature of normative political philosophy on democratic theory there are two broad traditions. In the first, often called the "interest group theory of democracy," the role of democratic political institutions is to provide a means of resolving the often conflicting interests of individuals and groups in the society in order to reach outcomes that maximally satisfy the overall interests of all members of the society.[13] In this theory, legislative representatives are properly responsive to interest groups in the society that they represent so long as all interests can be put on a relatively level playing field. Devices such as vote trading among representatives properly allow individuals to reflect differences in the intensity of their preferences or the strengths of their interests on different issues and to have a greater impact on issues that have more substantial effects on their interests. This version of democracy is commonly associated with preference satisfaction versions of utilitarian or consequentialist moral theories in which morally justified actions and public policies are those that maximally satisfy the desires or preferences of all affected by them. Individual citizens in this version of democracy are typically understood to be what Charles Taylor has called "weak evaluators."[14] The evaluations they express in their preferences and that they pursue in the push and pull of democratic decision making are essentially matters of taste. They are like preferences for different flavors of ice cream, for which no reason need be nor typically is given beyond the fact that one simply likes one particular flavor more than others.

Taylor contrasts weak evaluators and evaluations with strong evaluators and evaluations. Strong evaluations and preferences are backed by reasons that typically have a place in a person's broader evaluative framework or conception of a good life, of a good person, or of a just society; their importance is based on the role they play in that comprehensive moral or evaluative conception. Although there may be little to be said when two weak evaluators disagree about whether chocolate is better than vanilla—indeed they probably would not even think in terms of one being "better than" the other, as opposed simply to being liked more—the criticism and defense of strong evaluations is a matter of reasoning, reasoning about the broader moral or evaluative conception in which the particular evaluation finds a place. Rationing judgments, and in particular substantive positions on any of Daniels's rationing problems, are strong evaluations and so democratic procedures that address and resolve them must treat them not as mere preferences or interests to be aggregated, as with the interest-group theory, but as judgments or evaluations for reasoning and deliberation. This alternative conception of democracy, typically called deliberative democracy, understands the roles of citizens and/or their representatives to be common deliberation about the public good or interest and about justice.[15] The institutional task for the deliberative theory of democracy is to develop political institutions that foster this kind of deliberation in place of the pursuit of private interests typical in the interest group theory and in much of our actual politics. I shall draw from work on two distinct problems for beginning the task of characterizing the sort of procedures needed: first, an account of the process through which individuals can reach justified moral judgments; second, an account of the kinds of interests individuals have in fair democratic political processes for resolving their disagreements about justice.

The Justification of Moral Judgments

I begin with the justification of moral judgments. Suppose that a person's moral judgments are best understood as expressions of his or her attitudes and that there are no independent, objectively correct or true (or at least uncontroversially such) moral standards against which those judgments could be shown to be correct or mistaken. How can those judgments be justified? John Rawls has used the notion of considered moral judgments held in wide reflective equilibrium for the kind of process I have in mind.[16] Even if moral judgments are expressions of an individual's attitudes, they differ from mere matters of taste in that they are backed by reasons themselves part of a broader moral conception, and these reasons and moral conceptions can be critically evaluated.

Very briefly, the idea is this. We start at any point in time with the moral judgments that we accept and about which we have relatively high confidence or conviction. We then subject these judgments to what I think of as a critical screening process, attempting to avoid or correct for conditions that we know from experience lead to mistakes.[17] Many of these conditions will not be special to moral judgments, such as insufficient time to consider the question; lack of relevant information, ability, or expertise to evaluate it; being emotionally over-wrought, and so on. Other conditions may be special to moral judgments, such as when one's own interests will be importantly affected by the question at hand; then the worry is that we may rationalize in the pejorative sense by tailor-ing our judgments to serve our own interests in a manner that we would not accept from others.

Another part of this process is seeking to understand and to critically evalu-ate as fully as possible the nature of the moral reasons for a particular moral judgment or position. This will typically be done by beginning from a reason specific to the initial concrete case, considering its implications for other cases to which it applies and whether those implications are acceptable. When there are unacceptable implications of our initial judgments, we will have to clarify and sometimes revise or qualify those judgments and the reasons we offer for them. A further important part of this process is considering possible criticisms of our position on the case in question and of the moral reasons we have for that position. This involves considering any significant alternative positions that we might hold on the initial case in question and the acceptability of their implica-tions for other cases. This process often begins as an intrapersonal process, as we seek to think through a particular moral issue or case on our own. But it should also be an interpersonal process because we know from experience that others often have perspectives, criticisms, alternative positions, and arguments that we have missed or have not adequately considered.

As we engage in this critical screening process over time for different moral issues and cases, we will sometimes find inconsistencies among our moral judg-ments and reasons that will need to be resolved. Sometimes we do this by revis-ing or qualifying the moral reasons or principles to which we initially appealed, in other cases by revising our initial judgments on the issue or case with which we began. Because our degree of confidence in different concrete moral judg-ments and in more general moral reasons, principles, or comprehensive theories varies substantially, we will try to resolve inconsistencies by revising our initial moral views so as to leave us with overall moral views in which we have as much confidence as possible.

This is only a very brief summary that I and others have elaborated in much greater detail elsewhere of how people can critically evaluate their moral judg-ments, but several points bear emphasis.[18] First, our moral judgments that sur-vive in what Rawls called wide reflective equilibrium will be justified in the sense that they have survived a process of full critical scrutiny; they are what we believe after having considered as fully as possible all objections and alternatives to our initial moral judgments. Unlike moral realists who believe in objective moral truths that we can know to be true, in this account our judgments are not justified because they have been shown to be true by the realist's standards for moral truth. Second, the extent to which different individuals will hold the same moral views at the end of this process is an open empirical question; I believe there is no reason to expect full agreement or convergence and good reason to expect that people will tend to divide along the lines distinguishing familiar overall moral conceptions or theories. Third, I have sketched an ideal process of maximal critical evaluation, which in actual practice, of course, can only be more or less incompletely realized.

If this process yields a plausible account of justification for an individual's moral judgments, then we can use it as part of an answer to the democracy problem, specifically what would be fair democratic procedures for making justified and just rationing decisions. Those procedures should give us assurance that the moral judgments of individuals who participate in making the rationing decisions have been subjected to such a process of critical evaluation. It is the deliberative not the interest-group conception of democracy that has the resources we need. It understands democratic decision making as common and public deliberation about strong evaluations, backed by reasons that fit within broader moral conceptions of justice and the common good, not as simply a marketplace where citizens pursue their private interests. Fair democratic procedures that are appropriate for addressing rationing problems must dispose and direct their participants to approach rationing problems in terms of what would be fair or just, not simply what would serve their respective interests.

The critical screening process that I have just sketched for moral judgments generally, and rationing judgments in particular, provides an account of when individuals' moral judgments would be justified. But the rationing problems require a collective or social decision process that can be used by individuals whose justified considered moral judgments about how to ration are in conflict; more is needed than an account of justification for an individual's moral judgments. How should the relevant decision-making process be supplemented when we shift from an individual making up his or her mind about the rationing problems to individuals who have come to different conclusions in that process now having to reach collective agreement on them? The collective agreement they are seeking does not require that each individual arrive at the same moral judgments on the rationing problems—I am assuming that is typically not possible—but that they identify a collective decision process whose results all will accept as having been fairly arrived at given their individual differences.

Beitz's "Complex Proceduralism"

I have no complete answer to this question, and there would not be space here to detail a full answer in any case, but I will draw on work by Charles Beitz to at least sketch a promising direction for an account of the necessary fair procedures.[19] Beitz develops the notion of "complex proceduralism" for making social or political decisions such as rationing choices. Particular decision-making procedures will be justified to individuals on the basis of the specific interests those individuals have in what those procedures will be and in the decisions to be made with them. Beitz distinguishes two perspectives from which citizens of a democracy can view political institutions—as the "makers" of government and its policies and as the "matter" (i.e., the objects) of government and policy. Political institutions should be justifiable to citizens from both of these standpoints, and more specifically from the "regulative interests" that arise from both aspects of citizenship. Beitz proposes that individuals have three principal regulative interests in democratic decision procedures. "Recognition interests" concern "the terms on which citizens recognize each other as participants in public deliberation and choice";[20] they must express the democratic commitment to equal concern and respect for all citizens. Individuals' interest in "equitable treatment" requires that procedures not unnecessarily place the satisfaction of their needs and the success of their projects in jeopardy; it recognizes that we have substantive, not just procedural, notions of equity that apply to political institutions and decisions. Citizens' interest in "deliberative responsibility" requires that democratic institutions embody a commitment to resolution of political issues on the basis of public deliberation that is adequately informed, open to a wide range of competing views, and takes place in conditions in which these views can be reasonably assessed.

Political or social decision-making procedures will be fair, Beitz argues, if no one could reasonably reject them on the basis of his or her regulative interests. This does not define a unique decision-making process as fair but instead rules out some processes as unfair; for example, if they deny participation to a segment of the community, put some participants' basic liberties at risk, or resolve issues in private or only in terms of the parties' self-interest. Different decision-making procedures, even for specific kinds of decisions to be made in a specific social or political context, could satisfy Beitz's criterion of fairness, and if so any of them would be fair. A diverse array of possible fair procedures is especially likely for rationing decisions because, as noted earlier, in our complex and heterogeneous health care system, these decisions would have to be made in many quite different social and institutional contexts. Even with a more coherent national health care system, the rationing problems would require decisions at different levels or places within that system.

Whether Beitz's same regulative interests would govern decision-making procedures outside of the basic democratic political system is problematic, but I will assume that they would in order to pursue the example of a staff model HMO deciding about the priority of treatment for chronic schizophrenia versus treatment for mild to moderate OCD. What are the implications of Beitz's account of procedural fairness there? The recognition interest would require that coverage of treatments for these conditions not be decided, as it often is, by administrators of the HMO unilaterally or in negotiations about plan coverage between the HMO and the employers paying for members' health insurance costs. Plan members (subscribers) should have representatives with a full role in such decisions. The deliberative responsibility interest would require that decision making, and especially the reasons for particular rationing trade-offs, be open and available to all affected. More important and more difficult is ensuring that decisions are debated and made on principled grounds, not just in terms of the self-interest of potentially affected parties. For example, describing different states of disability in general, nondisease-specific terms, as opposed to explicit prioritizing of treatments for specific diseases such as schizophrenia versus OCD, can help shift the decision making from a clash of competing interest groups to a deliberation about articulated principles and judgments. Oregon used such general descriptions of limitations in function in its adaptation of Kaplan's Quality of Well-Being scale, including its prioritization of mental health services. The implications of the equitable treatment interest for health care rationing decisions are the least clear. I would interpret it as requiring some limits on the degree to which individuals' health care needs could be left unmet by fair rationing decisions. What is problematic is how that standard of minimal equity should be determined, because we want to use the decision-making procedures to set the limits on treatments to be provided. This is a deep and complex theoretical difficulty in any appeal to democratic procedures to arrive at solutions to problems of justice, but I cannot pursue it here. The best that may be possible in practice is to try to establish a consensus, based not on the decision-making procedure being developed but on an overlapping consensus among theories of justice and among citizens about what should be part of a minimal package of services or benefits; for example, in the case of schizophrenia that would require at least not leaving patients untreated and abandoned on the streets, as we have too often done in recent years.

This brief discussion of what might be fair decision-making procedures in one institutional context for addressing rationing problems barely begins the complex and controversial task of fully spelling out such procedures, much less putting them in place. I have only wanted to illustrate one possible structured approach for beginning to address what fair procedures might be within one institutional context in which rationing decisions could be made.

The Gap between Ideal and Real

I want to conclude by acknowledging the depressingly large gap between the kind of appeal to fair democratic procedures that could lay claim to resolving rationing problems justly and the typical political processes by which rationing and prioritization of mental health services are typically done. In real-world political struggles over mental health care budgets, priorities, or benefits coverage, there is too often little that comes close to the critical screening process to eliminate mistakes and prejudices in individuals' moral judgments and to subject them to criticism, together with a deliberative political process that satisfies individuals' interests in recognition, deliberative responsibility, and equitable treatment. Instead, the processes more typically lack any effective critical screening process and are deeply infected with prejudices and false beliefs about mental illness and its treatment in general, and about specific mental illnesses and treatments in particular, together with a political process that is closer to a conflict among self-interested partisans than common deliberation about just rationing. And the real-world alternative increasingly is unilateral decisions by large for-profit managed care plans driven by fierce competitive pressures to sign up new members and increase profits to satisfy the securities markets. These pressures were sufficiently intense in my former home state of Rhode Island to lead one of the largest national managed care corporations to erect such systematic and severe barriers to mental health care that the state Department of Health took the unprecedented step of temporarily suspending the operation of the organization managing its mental health care services and forcing the removal of its top management.

This gap between the ideal and the real may seem so wide as to make the theoretical worries about appeals to fair democratic procedures to settle disagreements about just rationing of mental health services, to which I have given most of my attention here, of little practical importance in any overall moral evaluation of real world prioritization and rationing of mental health services. I have considerable sympathy with this complaint. The most serious ethical concerns about the justice of many if not most actual decision-making processes to prioritize and ration mental health services are grosser ethical failures than the issues about the democracy problem on which I have concentrated here. Nevertheless, the issues that I have discussed are among the more important and difficult issues that I believe we face if we want to answer Daniels's democracy problem by justifying appeal to fair democratic procedures to resolve conflicts about how to prioritize and ration mental health services.

Notes

1. Norman Daniels, "Rationing Fairly," *Bioethics* 7, no. 2/3 (1993): 224–33, and reprinted (in part) as "Four Unsolved Rationing Problems: A Challenge," *Hastings Center Report* 24, no. 4 (1994): 27–29.

2. I discuss a few of the additional issues in "Some Unresolved Issues in Priority-Setting of Mental Health Services," in *What Price Mental Health? The Ethics and Politics of Setting Priorities*, ed. Philip Boyle and Daniel Callahan (Washington, D.C.: Georgetown University Press, 1995).

3. The most sophisticated and best treatment of some of these issues, though she develops some positions I do not share, is Frances Kamm, *Morality, Mortality*, vol. 1 (New York: Oxford University Press, 1993). For a statement of the early stage of work in normative ethical theory, see Derek Parfit, *Reasons and Persons* (Oxford: Oxford University Press, 1984), 3–4, 45.

4. Daniels has pursued some of these issues further in his recent book with James Sabin, *Setting Limits Fairly: Can We Learn to Share Medical Resources?* (Oxford: Oxford University Press, 2002).This article was completed before Daniels's and Sabin's book appeared and so does not take account of their work there on the democracy problem.

5. Dan W. Brock and Norman Daniels, "Ethical Foundations of the Clinton Administration's New Health Care System," *Journal of the American Medical Association* 271 (April 1994): 1189–96.

6. David Hadorn, "The Oregon Priority-Setting Exercise: Quality of Life and Public Policy," *Hastings Center Report* 21, no. 3 (May/June 1991): 11–16; David Eddy, "Oregon's Methods: Did Cost-Effectiveness Analysis Fail?" *Journal of the American Medical Association* 266, no. 21 (1991): 35–41.

7. Ronald Dworkin, *A Matter of Principle* (Cambridge, Mass.: Harvard University Press, 1985).

8. Daniels, "Rationing Fairly," 231.

9. John Rawls, *Theory of Justice* (Cambridge, Mass.: Harvard University Press, 1971).

10. Dan W. Brock, "Priority to the Worst Off in Health Care Resource Prioritization," in *Medicine and Social Justice*, ed. M. Battin, R. Rhodes, and A. Silver (New York: Oxford University Press, 2002).

11. Eric Nord, "The Trade-Off between Severity of Illness and Treatment Effect in Cost-Value Analysis of Health Care," *Health Policy* 24 (1993): 227–38.

12. Hadorn, "The Oregon Priority-Setting Exercise."

13. Robert A. Dahl, *Democracy and Its Critics* (New Haven, Conn.: Yale University Press, 1989).

14. Charles Taylor, "The Diversity of Goods," in *Utilitarianism and Beyond*, ed. Amartya Sen and Bernard Williams (Cambridge: Cambridge University Press, 1982).

15. Joshua Cohen, "Deliberation and Democratic Legitimacy," in *The Good Polity*, ed. D. Hamlin and P. Pettit (Oxford, England: Blackwell, 1991), 17–34; David Estlund, "Making Truth Safe for Democracy," in *The Idea of Democracy*, ed. D. Copp, J. Hampton, and J. Roemer (New York: Oxford University Press, 1983); Jon Elster, "The Market and the Forum," in *Foundations of Social Choice Theory*, ed. J. Elster and A. Hyliand (Cambridge: Cambridge University Press, 1986).

16. Rawls, *Theory of Justice*.

17. I have spelled out this idea of a critical screening process in more detail in "Public Moral Discourse," in *Society's Choices: Social and Ethical Decision Making in Biomedicine*, ed. Elizabeth Meyer Bobby, Harvey V. Fineberg, and Ruth E. Bulger (Washington, D.C.: National Academy Press, 1995).

18. Rawls, *Theory of Justice*, and Norman Daniels, "Wide Reflective Equilibrium and Theory Acceptance in Ethics," *Journal of Philosophy* 76, no. 5 (1979): 256–82.

19. See Charles R. Beitz, *Political Equality* (Princeton, N.J.: Princeton University Press 1989), ch.5. I am grateful to Norman Daniels for directing me to Beitz's treatment of fair procedures.

20. Beitz, *Political Equality*, 109.

CHAPTER 8

The Democracy Problem as Applied to the Oregon Health Plan and Its Prioritization of Mental Health Services

David A. Pollack

THIS CHAPTER DESCRIBES a real-life case example of prioritization or rationing in health care planning decisions and how that process can be understood to have dealt with the democracy problem as described by Norman Daniels[1] and clarified by Dan Brock.[2] The development and implementation of the Oregon Health Plan (OHP) is an appropriate natural experiment to evaluate whether and how the concerns about fair democratic procedures, procedural justice, and the balance between procedures and moral principles apply to practical public policy decisions.

I will first attempt to describe the elements of the OHP decision-making process throughout the course of the development of the prioritized list of conditions and their corresponding treatments. These descriptions will include the extent of representation in the various planning entities and other involved groups. I will also point out some of the factors that seemed to be influential in that process. This analysis will then review Brock's points about democracy and procedural justice, comparing his ideas about what constitutes a fair process with what seems to have happened in Oregon. I will conclude with several questions about how democracy may or may not work in making significant health policy decisions.

The Who and How of the Decisions

There were a number of decision-making bodies and other forms of input involved in various stages and with different aspects of the OHP planning process. During the prelegislative period, there were a number of attempts to gauge the public's interest in how health care decisions should be made and what were the most important priorities for scarce health care dollars. Most notable of these efforts were the activities of a highly influential public interest group, Oregon Health Decisions, which spearheaded the most organized activities of mobilizing and identifying public opinions on these issues. This group's efforts contributed significantly to the development of the collection of bills that eventually became the legislative foundation of the OHP. Indeed, many members on the board of Oregon Health Decisions, including the "father" of the OHP, John Kitzhaber, played important roles in the subsequent legislative process as well as the formal planning activities that the legislation mandated.

The original process that created the OHP in the 1989 session of the state legislature was certainly conducted in classical representative democratic fashion, whereby elected officials, with the help of various lobbying groups, crafted the laws that created the Health Services Commission (HSC) and the process for prioritizing or rationing services. Several lobbyists and the groups that they represented from the health and mental health community were very influential in this process.

Psychiatrists and other mental health professionals, consumers, and family advocates saw the need to come together to advocate for the needs of the mentally ill. They recognized that involvement in the decision-making process was essential if there was to be any hope of obtaining equity for persons who have mental disorders in relation to persons with other health conditions. This was especially true in view of the overwhelming history of stigma, discrimination, and disproportionately lower funds for services, provider compensation, or research. The influence of these citizens and lobbyists led to the inclusion of a special subcommittee of the HSC to address whether and how to include mental health and chemical dependency conditions and services in the overall health benefit package that the HSC was expected to design.

The HSC, appointed by the governor, was composed predominantly of persons who represented the health community, but included some representation of the general public. The Mental Health and Chemical Dependency (MHCD) subcommittee included providers, administrators, family advocates, and consumers from the mental health community. The HSC and its subcommittees operated in a very open fashion, allowed input from anyone who attended their meetings, and established methods for obtaining public opinion on many different issues about which they were making decisions. The decision-making process within the subcommittees was most often consensual and occasionally required votes to resolve conflicts. Some of the prioritization decisions involved more sophisticated approaches to rank-ordering categories of services and conditions, such as relative weights and Delphi decision methods.

Some of the methods to obtain public opinion included:

- a phone survey to obtain input regarding the relative value of different types of symptoms and impairments, the data of which were used in the Health Outcomes subcommittee's prioritization methodology;

- community meetings held throughout the state to provide education and obtain opinions on some of the values that should be used in making the prioritization decisions;
- public hearings conducted for the purpose of giving individuals and interest groups the opportunity to share their concerns about what was most important to them.

Although some of these opinion gathering methods have been criticized for having a skewed or unbalanced representation from the general public, genuine and concerted efforts were made to attract geographically, culturally, and economically diverse input. The relative weight and influence of the public opinion activities are very hard to gauge. There is no doubt, however, that the prevailing values and issues expressed were either incorporated into scientific data used to rank conditions and services or considered by members of the HSC subcommittees when they made their subjective prioritization decisions.

As the planning process progressed, an unprecedented mental health coalition, including representatives from professional and provider groups, family advocates, and consumers, formed to oversee and attempt to influence the planning process. This group agreed to set aside many previously intense turf and philosophical conflicts in order to pursue the superordinate goal of obtaining parity coverage for persons with mental disorders. This group contributed many ideas and much data to the MHCD subcommittee, including the submission of people as candidates for membership on the subcommittee (and for later appointments to other planning and oversight bodies).

Finally, there were the various groups of public officials who were charged with participating in the process as staff, data providers, or regulators. These included numerous state agency representatives, especially from the state offices or departments of Medicaid, Health, Mental Health, and Alcohol and Drug services. Some of these state officials were directly involved and very invested in the processes working successfully. Others were more skeptical, especially if they interpreted the process as unlikely to succeed or threatening to their particular sphere of influence, and they resisted efforts to obtain their help.

The other major influence was from the federal officials and other out-of-state special-interest groups who were concerned with the state's project and its compliance with various Medicaid regulations. The process of obtaining the federal Medicaid waiver for the OHP project was contaminated by political factors, not the least of which was that of the 1992 presidential election and the fear expressed by organizations representing various disadvantaged groups that the OHP would further discriminate against those who deserved entitlements or special protections. At one point, the Health Care Financing Administration (HCFA) waiver was threatened on the alleged basis of the OHP's not being fair to disabled persons. This was especially odd because most of the groups involved with those special populations within the state (including the mental health community) supported the OHP and were convinced that the prioritization process would reverse some of the discrimination that their constituents had experienced.

Influential Factors

Several relatively nonquantifiable factors played important roles but varied in their influence over the decision-making process. The differences in the composition of the various groups involved were very significant. Those groups composed of people directly involved in mental health care and who were most familiar with the local issues within the state initially struggled a great deal over the enormity of the process and the overwhelming implications of the decisions they were asked to make, not to mention the short amount of time they were allowed to make those decisions. At the same time, they saw themselves as involved in a very noble, forward-looking, and constructive effort, especially if it were to be successful. They were gratified that their experience and values were being included.

The relative level of activity of various participants, their fervor or stamina, and their ability to tolerate frustration and ambiguity contributed to whether certain individuals had significantly more influence than others. Some of the consumer participants dropped out or deferred to others who had more clinical expertise. Some advocates who had specified issues about which they were particularly concerned reduced their involvement after their issues had been addressed or if their advocacy seemed to provoke a more persuasive counterargument to their desired position. The combination of long meetings and complicated subject matter proved to be daunting for some participants, thus leading to attrition in some stages of the process and concentrating the decision-making power into a smaller number of hands.

Differential motivation and changes in the interest of participants certainly affected who elected to participate in some of the decision-making groups or the public opinion efforts. There were clearly some individuals who, because of their interest, persuasiveness, and other personality characteristics, were substantially more influential than others.

Analysis of the Democratic Process in Oregon

Brock's consideration of the democracy problem focuses on three particular aspects of the democratic process: the complexity of the democratic process, the limits to democratic procedures, and the danger that democratic preferences may be prejudicial, unscientific, or unlikely to have a positive outcome. The likelihood and necessity for multiple inputs reflect the complexity of democratic processes and the need for decision-making bodies to be disaggregated. Limits to democratic procedures include risk of veto, constitutional constraints, administrative costs, or time limits.

Brock describes the concept of "imperfect procedural justice" as a probably realistic notion of how decisions can and will be made, in view of the impossibility of obtaining a flawless democratic process. This concept is associated with the notion that independent standards and "fair" procedures are disputable and unsettled and that there is a sufficient amount of indeterminacy, depending on the participant's perspective, to lead to a reliance on procedures to resolve or reconcile them.

He goes on to describe lines of defense for justifying the use of procedures. They must involve "considered moral judgments," which put the procedures through a relevant and plausible critical screening process to determine whether they are justified. It is important to obtain consensual validation through "wide reflective equilibrium" by running the judgments past a representative group of participants who would have to live with the results of the process. Fair political processes or "political equality" must also somehow be demonstrated by having significant participation (even if it is through representatives), equitable treatment of the subjects of the decision, and deliberative responsibility on the part of the decision makers. Fairness is achieved if the results cannot be rejected on the basis of any of these factors. Others have described fairness as being a combination of the following ingredients: ownership of the decision by the decision-making body, transparency of the decision-making process, and identification of the need as collective or communitarian, not parochial.

How does the process of prioritization planning for the OHP and the inclusion of mental health conditions measure up to these standards? In spite of Brock's and others' pessimism about fairness in general and the risks of concentrating decision-making power too much, especially in the hands of groups whose vested interest is overtly in conflict with their considered responsibility (such as unscrupulous managed care companies in Rhode Island that excessively deny services to those who truly need them), the process in Oregon appears to have been conforming to and continues to conform to many of Brock's articulated principles of fair democratic procedures.

There was reasonably wide participation by people throughout the state from a wide range of special interests, including general citizens as well as experts, in many of the arenas of decision making and data gathering. The prioritization process involved a fair balance between the reliance on intuitive or theoretically based judgments and expressed preferences by participants. There were both "weak" and "strong" evaluators. There was a balance between the use of procedures and the persuasion of moral principles. This was accomplished in part by having a long series of meetings in which the participants grew to know and respect one another, which gave the opportunity for individuals to question the majority's apparent position on some issues. One of the specific benefits to MHCD services from this process was that we were helped to overcome certain biased views and to debunk the false dichotomous notion of the separation of mind and body. Some of the procedures involved our being blind to the opinions of others until those opinions were expressed and then discussing them at some length with the hope of arriving at compromise or some other form of conflict resolution. The amount of education that was promoted regarding the importance of MHCD conditions, the effectiveness of treatments for those conditions, and the comparability of MHCD conditions to other health care concerns all helped to reduce the risk of prejudice or false belief contaminating the decision process. Throughout the process, various participants reminded the larger groups of the need to adhere to "what would be just, not what would serve their respective interests."

The imperfect procedures used to make decisions were sufficiently fair or adequate ("good enough") to be acceptable to all of the participants. These procedures depended on data that were provided from a wide array of sources and included reasonable methods for resolving indeterminacy (however, in some instances when indeterminacy could not be overcome, certain decisions were delayed or resolved in a more limited way). In any case, many differences of opinion were resolved by the appeal to procedures and the deliberative process in which considered moral judgments were often held in reflective equilibrium (albeit briefly at times). The prioritization decisions went through several screens of critical (some would say hypercritical) scrutiny before being fully approved. In most instances, broader moral conceptions of justice took precedence over or were appealed to in order to transcend private or special interests.

Lingering Questions

In spite of the apparent sufficiency of fairness and democracy in the Oregon process, a number of theoretical issues and questions remain. The answers to these questions are likely to be very difficult to establish, but essential in order to confidently proceed with similar planning efforts on a larger scale.

- How legitimate is democracy-by-extension (via experts and stakeholders) or representative democracy (via elected or appointed officials) in arriving at "fair" decisions?
- How effective and fair is it to use education of selected groups or the general public to influence policy decisions?
- Is it fair for those who stick with the process (because of stamina, longevity, or tenacity) to have a relatively greater influence over the decisions?

- Leadership qualities (charisma, compelling ideas, credentials) in certain individuals can affect the group's decisions. Does this contaminate the process?
- Is a certain minimum level of expertise necessary to make these very important, and sometimes quite technical, decisions?
- Is it appropriate to secure and use safeguards against unacceptable but democratically derived decisions? Is there justification for a deciding group's insistence that certain decisions be protected from public influence or notification?
- How important and influential is or should be the strategic development of consensus among associated but competitive groups in achieving influence over the ultimate decision? If such previously disparate entities can agree on a recommendation, shouldn't that agreement carry significant weight?
- Is the appearance of democracy more important than the reality of democratic process if the ultimate decision is seen to be good or fair?
- As with the notion of the "good enough" mother or parent, what constitutes a fair enough decision process?

In Oregon, we didn't have the luxury of unlimited amounts of time or resources to make the prioritization decisions. We did have dedicated groups of participants who made a good-faith effort to be honest and fair in the process. In retrospect and in comparison with the process for deciding how to deliver mental health services in some other states (Tennessee, Rhode Island, New York, and Florida) we may have done as fair a job as is practically conceivable. The outcomes of this experiment will ultimately determine the answers to these questions. The process we went through, however, was valuable for all of us, within and outside of the state, in demonstrating how to practically apply a number of very challenging and ennobling ideas about how to make tough but fair decisions.

Notes

1. Norman Daniels, "Rationing Fairly: Programmatic Considerations," *Bioethics* 7, nos. 2/3 (1993): 224–33.
2. See Dan Brock, "The Democracy Problem in Mental Health Care Priority Setting," chapter 7 in this book.

CHAPTER 9

Saving the Worst Off (Principle)

James Lindemann Nelson

MY AIM HERE is to explore and defuse—or at least deflect—a number of challenges that need to be answered if a principle prescribing some degree of *preference for the worst off* (also referred to here as prioritarianism) is to be recognized as a useful tool for guiding allocation decisions in mental health care.[1] That those who are "worst off" should have some kind of special claim on scarce resources strikes many people as intuitively plausible, and it has been incorporated into sophisticated discussions of distributive justice, perhaps most notably in the hands of John Rawls,[2] Frances Kamm,[3] and Amartya Sen.[4] But preferring the worst off also seems plainly incompatible with highly developed understandings of what justice bids us do, and, just as plainly, prioritarianism suffers considerable interpretive problems of scope and stringency.

As it strikes me, the attractiveness of assigning priority to the worst off is most clearly displayed by tracing its relationship to basic moral intuitions—perhaps primarily to the surely plausible notion that it is at least prima facie unjust to give *more still* to those who already have more at the expense of those who have less. The Aristotelian idea that justice is about "some kind" of equality also seems pertinent, as preferring the worst off appears a reasonable way of achieving equality of the right kind.[5] Furthermore, despite the fact that prioritarianism is typically thought to be an anticonsequentialist principle, support for the worst-off preference can be found in the utilitarian-flavored idea of "decreasing marginal value"; the thought here is that the same amount of goods will do less to enhance the welfare of those who already have more goods than it will to those who have less.

In a recent essay, Dan Brock has carefully surveyed these and other possible justifications for assigning priority to the worst off.[6] In addition to the considerations already outlined, he notes that contractualist moral theorists such as Thomas Scanlon and Thomas Nagel focus their attention on the seriousness of complaints that individuals can urge on their own behalf, contrasted with complaints of other individuals. The aim of distributive justice in their view is to minimize the complaints of those whose complaints are the gravest, and a natural interpretation of this aim is to see the worst off as those with the gravest complaints.

Thus, there are readily available "nonconsequentialist," "consequentialist," and "contractualist" forms of backing for the worst-off principle. However, the idea that a policy of preference for the worst off should dominate or even strongly influence deliberations concerning resources allocation is also contested on many grounds, both broadly consequentialist and nonconsequentialist. It is insofar as these criticisms try to show that prioritarianism is not relevant to questions of distributive justice that I try to rebut them.

I start by considering large-scale, theoretical challenges; these allege that preference for the worst off is in principle an inappropriate aim of allocation policy, as it conflicts with directives that emerge from better supported moral theories. The chief critics here are familiar forms of utilitarianism, but I will also consider Eric Rakowski's nonconsequentialist theory of justice. Next, I turn to apparently counterintuitive implications of preferring the worst off: for example, that doing so discourages a primary care orientation in health care contexts or that it may tend too indiscriminately to favor the elderly over the young, at least in the distribution of resources not aimed at extending life. I then take up the concern that preference for the worst off must be defined in an arbitrarily restrictive way if it is to guide allocation. The worry here is that people are seldom simply patients with mental health problems; many other dimensions of their lives contribute to their being either worse off or better off than other people. Finally, I will discuss some matters having to do with setting preferences for the worst off into balance with other relevant goals of mental health policy, such as maximizing overall benefit and (other dimensions of) fairness.

Addressing this last task adequately would involve answering the crucial question of just how much priority the worst off should receive. I do not pretend to have achieved much toward a convincing answer to that question here. Indeed, I'm inclined to think that the best it is reasonable for us to expect from moral theorizing is a fairly complete and perhaps roughly "weighted" overview of all the considerations that are relevant to allocation decisions so that our deliberations are not missing important considerations. I do not live in the hope of the advent of a convincing algorithm. There is, however, a fair amount of ground that needs to be cleared before we can have good reason to think that the priority principle can lay claim to an important place at the distributive table and hence that what is left unresolved here is worth the effort to try to sort out elsewhere.

Challenges from Theory

Utilitarianism

Utilitarianism prescribes choosing actions or policies that will achieve the most favorable balance of good over bad consequences (for some specification of "good" and "bad") and thus would seem to yield a straightforward theory-based objection to giving priority to the worst off. Preferring the worst off *might*, of course, have optimal results in those circumstances where the goods to be handed out diminish sharply in relative value according to how much of those goods potential recipients already enjoy. But without evidence supporting that such circumstances actually obtain across the board (or, for present purposes, within mental health), it seems implausible to see favoring the worst off as a reliable way of doing the most to achieve any of the standard conception of the good—pleasure, happiness, preference satisfaction, and so on—that utilitarians target. It certainly looks as though other candidates for guiding allocation decisions—for example, "favor those who will be most responsive to treatment," or "prefer treatments that will make the most patients fully functional"—would seem more likely to produce the most "good," at least granted certain plausible empirical assumptions.

If, for example, patients who were severely mentally ill could achieve marginal gains for the same expenditure as would allow moderately mentally ill people to achieve near-normality, then the only way a utilitarian would be able to favor the worst off is if there were an enormous number of the severely ill who could be helped with the available resources or if the benefits of small functional gains were much more productive of good to the severely ill than the attainment of near-normality would be to the moderately ill. But, as Frances Kamm has noted, there are widely shared intuitions to the contrary, expressing the sense that attaining psychological normality represents a much more significant good to a mentally ill person than would any gains that leave a person substantially short of normality, even if the relative improvement in function seemed in some respects greater for those left short.[7]

Kamm's point might be seen as redirecting our understanding of what counts as being worse off in these contexts. As a minimal interpretation, the priority principle dictates that given that roughly equal degrees of improvement are attainable, scarce resources should be directed to those who are worse off from the start. But if the achievement of normality represents a good distinct in character and higher in value than functional improvements that fall short of normality, then those who are capable of attaining that good given the provision of the resources, it might be thought, are now in a different position vis-à-vis their less functional competitors for the resource. They are more badly off for the lack of the good that will normalize them than are those who, although functionally less able at the start, cannot attain normality if they receive the resource.

Although I'm not suggesting that Kamm would see the matter this way herself, it does seem quite clear that standard-issue utilitarians would not be able to take advantage of this strategy for accommodating the intuition that normality is of special value. Therefore, a utilitarian approach cannot account both for this intuition and for the priority principle as well. The idea that psychological normality represents a special kind of good makes sense in a context that recognizes qualitatively distinct kinds of goods: the "special kind of good" point cannot be reduced to the notion that those normalized are likely to be happier or have a better ratio of satisfied to unsatisfied preferences than nonnormal people made functionally better off by the intervention. Indeed just the opposite might well be the case.

The inability to account for different kinds of value seems to me one of the primary reasons why utilitarianism cannot make much sense of giving priority to the worst off, as well as one of the primary reasons why utilitarianism as such is implausible.

There are, of course, others. The discussion generated by considering the pros and cons of variants on utilitarian themes as an ethical theory or even as a theory of social policy formation is, of course, far too voluminous to do much more than gesture in its general direction. It is a commonplace that utilitarianism violates many moral intuitions that are both widely shared and deeply ingrained; although some utilitarians have attempted to square variants of their approach with the greatest part of such intuitions, others have allowed that utilitarianism ought not to be assessed by its fidelity to general beliefs about morality, no matter how widely shared or clearly and consistently arrayed. Rather, it should be seen as a rational replacement of the systems of taboos that have previously passed for moral systems.

However, critical work by John Rawls and Bernard Williams, inter alia, suggests that utilitarianism violates not just moral beliefs that we may happen to share but something even deeper—our sense of ourselves as distinct agents. Rawls has pointed out that "utilitarianism does not take seriously the distinction between persons,"[8] and Williams has expanded this insight in arguing that utilitarianism is incompatible with personal integrity.

Noting that the identities of human beings are caught up in a special way with certain of their "projects," "attitudes," or "commitments," Williams has pointed out that utilitarianism demands that we think of our relationship to those projects as a matter of how their pursuit meshes with "the utility network which the projects of others have in part determined."[9] Such a way of regarding our projects alienates us from our "actions and the source of [our] actions in [our] own convictions." It is insensitive to the extent to which identifying actions and decisions as our own is a function of those acts and choices stemming from the projects and attitudes with which we are most identified. In dismissing the importance of this identification, utilitarianism is, "in the most literal sense,"[10] an attack on our integrity. Thus the price of accepting a utilitarian orientation is not merely resigning what may be deeply held moral beliefs; it costs us our sense of ourselves as distinct agents. This is not so much moral revisionism as it is a wholesale replacement of the underpinnings of the thoughts and practices against which the backdrop of moral reasoning makes sense.[11]

This criticism can be understood as an effort to reveal just how deeply resistance to an altogether aggregative approach to moral reasoning is rooted, and it is in large part as an aggregative theory that utilitarianism will resist prioritarianism. However, one could imagine a form of consequentialist approach to mental health care rationing that would, in effect, compare individuals and their possible gains in a pairwise fashion. If Jane were more severely mentally ill than George, but if the best available interventions will make her only marginally better, whereas George would make substantial gains from the best intervention that could be offered him, then a policy that ranked underwriting treatment for those in George's position higher than underwriting treatment for those in Jane's position could be defended against the charge of not taking individuals with due seriousness.

Yet this nonaggregative consequentialism cannot make clear sense out of the idea that, apart from differences in the subjective impact of the magnitude of the improvement available, anyone could be so situated that her *need* for improvement makes a more stringent moral demand on us than does anyone else's. Again, ignoring differences in need might seem to many counterintuitive, but, as in the earlier criticism of more standard utilitarianisms, it is inviting to try to clear a higher bar by pointing out discordances between consequentialism and settled features of our conceptual practices. Consider this: seeing "magnitude of improvement" as a consideration that always serves as *the* reason for making distributive decisions is to credit it with a very unusual kind of property. As Jonathan Dancy has pointed out, in both theoretical and practical contexts, what counts as a reason for belief or for action will typically be *holistic*— that is, sensitive to the context in which a consideration obtains. If a stick looks bent, that is in general a good reason for believing that it is bent—but not if the stick is half in the water. Or, as Dancy says about practical reasons, "that there will be nobody much else there is sometimes a good reason for going there, and sometimes a very good reason for staying away."[12] Although considerations of the holism of reasons do not show that priority for the worse off should be recognized as an independent and significant factor in decisions about distributing scarce resources, it does undermine another one of the characteristic features of consequentialist approaches that is incompatible with prioritarianism.

It might be tempting to think that reason holism would be just as damaging to the aspirations of prioritarianism as to consequentialist approaches, but on reflection, this criticism is not plausible. Priority to the worst off need not be seen as dominating distributive discourse to have a significant role in shaping it, and holism does not imply that certain considerations may not be *more or less* stable as useful guides to morally defensible action. That is all that is being urged for giving priority to the worst off at present.

Eric Rakowski's Prudent Insurer Approach

Although the Williams style of objection to utilitarianism—in brief, that it illicitly uses decision principles appropriate for one-person cases in many-person cases and thus neglects the separateness of persons—is not without its critics,[13] I regard it as well taken, and (taking due account of the effectiveness of the holism of practical reasoning in undermining less aggressively aggregative consequentialism as well) I will proceed as if assigning priority to the worst off has nothing mortal to fear from a utilitarian quarter. Yet Eric Rakowski's theory of distributive justice, although not utilitarian, does suggest that a first-person point of view is the appropriate stance to take in designing policy concerning allocation of health care resources. Although Rakowski does not advocate aggregating the preferences of the many into one sum, he does claim that, apart from unusual instances that might confront individuals having to decide how to allocate their own resources to aid others, the worst-off problem does not arise.[14] Figuring out whether to and how much to privilege the worst off is not a problem that would need to be solved as an issue of system design.

I understand Rakowski's position like so: individuals should have access to those resources needed to make what strikes them as prudent insurance decisions protecting them against future misfortune. Moral and technical problems must be addressed by this view, but deciding whether and what preference should be extended to the worst off is not among them; ideally, how the worst off would fare (and who they would be) would be settled by the insurance decisions that people actually made, decisions that would not involve reflection on the worst off.

It seems to me that this view sidesteps the worst-off problem by relying on the assumption that only morality and not prudence must take the problem seriously. This assumption is unargued and, as I think, not self-evidently true. Making decisions for our own futures is a clear case of decision making under uncertainty, just the kind of situation for which maximin strategies are taken to be apt, at least if certain other conditions are met. But maximin decision strategies, in counseling us to avoid the worst alternatives, imply that we should adopt policies designed to make our worst possible futures as good as possible. This is analogous, in the order of prudence, to accepting a preference for the worst-off principle in the order of morality.

The following conditions are taken to make maximin a reasonable approach in general:

1. There must be reason to sharply discount estimates of the differing probability of various future contingencies.
2. The conception of the good held by the person choosing is such that she cares little for what might be gained over and above that which is ensured by adopting a preference for the worst off.
3. The worst possible situations are unacceptable.[15]

Rawls tells us that, to the extent that these conditions are met, maximin is an appropriate rule for decision making under uncertainty.[16] Are these conditions met in the sort of decisions that face Rakowski's prudent insurers as they consider what kind of mental health coverage they will elect? The answer is no and yes. If not all, surely *some* decision makers will find themselves in a position where these conditions are satisfied to a considerable degree. Many will have a conception of the good such that ill-treated severe and persistent mental illness is regarded as unacceptable, motivating a "sharp discount" for estimates of the changes of succumbing (about 5.4 percent of the population acquires severe mental illness in any given year).[17] Thus the kinds of goods to which they might have greater access if they did not heavily insure against the worst possibilities—say, greater access to counseling for marital problems or other "problems in living"—strike them as comparatively inconsequential. There seems nothing at all implausible in many people's having this constellation of beliefs and preferences. Thus, strictly from the point of view of wanting their own lives to go overall as well as possible, rationality would seem to direct such people at least to consider carefully the weight a first-person version of the worst-off problem should play in their decision making.

If this is correct, then at least many people deliberating about their futures need to consider precisely the issues on the table here if they are to be rational. Although a canonical answer to the problem would not be incorporated into the design of a Rakowski-style allocation plan, because the direction of resources would lie in the hands of individuals, there would seem to be a social responsibility to be sure the matter was well aired so that individual decision makers would enjoy the best possible chance of making rational decisions. Among the resources that people need to make prudent insurance decisions may include a presentation of relevant conceptual as well as empirical information. This would seem to include promulgating widely, in suitable forms, the (no doubt various) results of philosophical deliberation on the issue.

One might make a stronger claim. Suppose we questioned the understanding of prudence that seems to be operating here and instead maintained that we have *moral* responsibilities to our future selves. Were this the case, it would be reasonable to think that any moral reasons we would have for taking seriously considerations of comparative disadvantage with respect to others we also have with respect to later stages of ourselves.

This view might seem particularly plausible in respect to mental health. If the persistence of personal identity over time has much to do with psychological continuity, then in making decisions about insuring for possible future schizophrenia, for example, I am in effect making a decision about someone whose relationship to me is not altogether a matter of strict numerical identity and so with respect to whom I am not authorized simply to accept whatever risks might fall within my own current conception of the good. (On this account, using decision principles appropriate for one-person cases might be inappropriate even in what are ostensibly one-person cases.)[18]

Of course, something might have to be said to show why I should regard myself as having any particular responsibility for any such "successor self." But whatever the right account of personal identity is, it is reasonable to think that many of my decisions in the present have uniquely significant implications for my future, or the future of my successor, and Rakowski's approach only adds to their number. For example, if we take Williams's notion of personal integrity seriously—seeing identity as at least in part a function of the kind of projects, commitments, and attitudes we take up—certain devastating forms of mental illness will clearly rupture our relationship with those endeavors and stances. At this point in time, then, I face the possibility of standing in a unique causal relationship to a person who is very badly off. This person is too distinct from me to regard her as covered by first-person prudential considerations but close enough for me to have a special responsibility for her just treatment—what her life will be like will depend upon decisions made now by me.

Although it surely complicates matters that the "worst off future state of ourselves (or of our successors)" is not an actual but merely a possible future state, *all* the states we are insuring against are merely possible: giving special attention to the worst-off state does not seem inappropriate simply because its future reality is not ensured.

To push this a bit farther, consider that reasons that might be given for a policy of preference for the worst off have what are at least close analogs when we reflect on the situation that a person faces while making decisions concerning how she will provide for possible futures. Consider the fairness argument: we should prefer the worst off over the less badly off, because otherwise those who are already better off than the worst off will be made better off still. If I consider possible future states and make decisions that will be to my advantage in those possible futures in which I am mildly depressed at the expense of those in which I am floridly psychotic, I am in effect already making better off possible future states of myself still better off than worse-off states. It is true that the agent deciding for herself will not be allocating resources between two currently needy individuals, but she might be likened to someone making health policy for a population whose members may be afflicted by a serious disease or by a lesser disease or both or neither. In allocating resources preferentially to the worst off on grounds of fairness, it does not seem essential that the planner know that certain people are in fact being afflicted by the serious illness; we do, after all, insure against occurrences that are not likely to occur but which would have devastating consequences.

Consider the diminishing marginal values argument. It can be argued that directing extra resources to the worst off is reasonable because those same resources will often translate into different and better kinds of goods for those who are worse off than for those who are better off. If it is reasonable to believe this in general regarding decision making affecting other people living at the same time, it would seem reasonable to believe it for possible future states of self. This conclusion is most defensible when a person is in a state of genuine uncertainty about her future or when she has reason to believe that her odds of depression versus psychosis are in the same neighborhood. If she has good reason to believe otherwise, she may not allocate resources strictly to possible worst-off futures in exclusion to better-off and more probable futures, but this does not entail that no preference for the worst off is appropriate here—only that other considerations are also relevant in the allocation of scarce resources.

Finally, consider the notion that the goal of justice is to reduce the complaints of those whose complaints are the most serious. If I think about states of my own life or about the life of those for whom I have a special responsibility it certainly seems plausible to say that those states or individuals that would be the worst off would have the gravest complaints against me now for not having made insurance decisions that would lessen their complaints.

Hence even if my aim for my life is simply that things go as well for me overall as possible, some preference for possible worst-off states of my future life seems appropriate. If I think it is possible to treat myself (or my "successors") more or less justly, extending such preference may be as morally incumbent on me in respecting myself as it is in respecting others. It may also be necessary, then, to set preferences for the worst off in equitable balance with other morally relevant concerns such as maximizing overall gain or achieving normality.

There are reasons, then, of both prudence and morality to doubt the notion that a prudent insurer approach to health care allocation makes careful consideration of the worst-off issue beside the point.

Intuitive Challenges

However, there are also grounds for believing that preference for the worst off—at least if it is at all a robust preference and not simply on the order of a tiebreaker of last resort—will conflict with widely shared and reasonable moral intuitions. Consider the following case.

Community mental health organizations have often been criticized for spending inappropriately on the problems of the "worried well"—counseling for lifestyle issues, marriage counseling, and such—rather than devoting resources to the severely and persistently ill.[19] Suppose it were the case, however, that some severe mental illnesses could be screened for and detected when they were asymptomatic and that expensive interventions were possible that would head off the full-blown emergence of the illness. Suppose further that the screening and subsequent interventions cost roughly the same as long-term treatment of those already ill from this disease. It is arguable that preventing illness is to be preferred, all else equal, to curing illness, because it avoids the kinds of disruptions in life that serious illness cause, even if they are later cured. It could well seem reasonable to privilege prevention in allocation for research and therapy. But those who have not yet suffered the effects of serious illness are clearly not among the worst off with respect to that illness; on the worst-off principle, it would seem more defensible to devote available resources to treating those who are already severely ill, even if it is not possible to restore them to full health, rather than to devote resources to preventing the occurrence of disease in those prone to it.

Here is a possible response. Although there is in general good moral reason to prefer prevention to cure, those reasons are not powerful enough to permit us to sink all our resources into prevention: despite our best efforts, many people—perhaps virtually everyone—will fall ill at some point, and, besides, we have not expended our best efforts in this direction. Further, there are some illnesses for which effective prevention is not available. It is rational then for us to put aside some of our resources to cure diseases, and among those afflicted by disease, the worst off should enjoy some preference, other things being equal. The worst-off principle, on this account, should not be used to compare those who are not yet ill with those who are, but rather those who suffer from some form of illness with other sufferers. Indeed, this is only one of the respects in which the scope of worst-off comparisons may need to be restricted; I will discuss this further in the following discussion.

Next, consider the case of intergenerational conflict. Suppose clozapine could be used to effectively cure a twenty-year-old schizophrenic in the first year of her illness, or a sixty-year-old schizophrenic in the thirty-first year, but not both. The elderly person could reasonably be said to be worse off. Should she therefore receive the clozapine?

In her discussion of the worst-off problem, Frances Kamm has distinguished between the dimension of need and the dimension of urgency; roughly, need is a matter of the character of one's experience overall considered as a function of lacking a benefit, whereas urgency concerns how much suffering will occur from this moment forth for lack of the benefit. (Urgency can in turn be analyzed into urgency^T—how soon one will be badly off for lack of the benefit—and urgency^Q—how badly off one will be soon for lack of the benefit.)[20] Kamm argued that, in contexts where life*saving* goods are being allocated, need is particularly significant and that those who have already lived longer should have less claim than those who have lived a shorter time, as the elder person has had more of the relevant good already and hence is less needy.[21] But if we are allocating a life-*enhancing* good, it would seem that those who have suffered longer with the illness are to that extent worse off and hence should have priority. The worst-off principle, then, seems to generate a preference for the elderly (or, more precisely, the long-suffering) when it comes to interventions designed to enhance life but a preference for the young when it comes to interventions designed to lengthen life. Because enhancing life by curing a serious illness in a young person might well also involve extending such a person's life, it might be thought that these preferences would yield odd or even incoherent policies. On the other hand, it might strike us that the principle is insightful here: the short-lived do have a greater claim on more life, the long-suffering have a greater claim on less suffering. The fact that ending suffering might have an impact on length of life could be accounted for by regarding the primary impact of the intervention with more seriousness than any collateral effects.

The Alleged Arbitrariness of Preference for the Worst Off

Some comparisons of how people are faring are reasonably straightforward. If I am schizophrenic and you are mildly depressed, I am clearly worse off than you. Other comparisons are harder. Imagine comparing someone who is moderately depressed with someone who has a moderately intense obsessive-compulsive disorder. Imagine further that different degrees of social support can have an impact on the subjective experience and degree of function related to these conditions. If this is the case, we should have to examine such things as family structures in order to make reasonable judgments of who is the worst off.

Suppose Mr. Close-Knit were functioning reasonably well due to a supportive family but not so well as he would were family care supplemented with intensive therapy. Suppose Ms. Functional is doing less well, in part because her family is not at all supportive. Ms. Functional seems less well off and therefore should have an advantage in competition for scarce therapeutic resources. These resources will make her considerably better off than Mr. Close-Knit will be. If his family, on having the allocation decision explained to them, were to say, "This only shows that no good deed goes unpunished" and informed the treatment team of their intention to immediately abandon their relative in order that he might become sick enough to compete realistically for curative interventions, would he then become poorly enough off to receive the relevant therapy? Or would the consequences of his abandonment be an "irrelevant disutility"? If such considerations as family background are relevant when they directly affect the experience of disease, why should they not be relevant when they affect other significant features of a person's life? Why should not income, quality of home life, and social standing all be used to determine differential degrees of how well or poorly off a person is? It would seem that they certainly connect with considerations of fairness, equality, marginal utility, and marginal value, the considerations that purport to undergird our acknowledgment of the special status of the worst off.

A natural reply is that in making allocation decisions concerning a certain kind of scarce good, one should regard the reason guiding the decision making to be how badly off one is with respect to that good. Thus a poor person with bipolar disease is not, in relevant respects, less well off than a rich person with bipolar disease. What is needed to support this claim is an argument to the effect that limiting the scope of the judgment of how different claimants are doing in this respect is not arbitrary. One possible such argument would allege that medical interventions seek to do good or forestall what is bad in certain respects—roughly, in respects that concern how bodies function and that express themselves in terms of interference with adequate conscious life—and that it is only considerations concerning those respects that are relevant to determinations of who is more or less badly off with respect to medical goods.

Is this an adequate reply? Kamm connects it to a Walzerian "spheres of justice" approach, which asserts that different regions of human activity and value acquire distinct sorts of social meaning; the goods in those spheres cluster together. Medicine's sphere involves such matters as health and disease, not (for example) economic distribution.[22]

This reply does not seem to me to dispel altogether the concern about arbitrary limitations. It suggests either that medicine has a natural telos that somehow makes it inappropriate to think of its possible impacts on other dimensions of human life, which seems implausible, or that the "social meanings" assigned to medicine are not open to critical scrutiny and revision, which I find also implausible.[23] Neither, however, does it seem altogether without force. The comparative judgment "X is worse off than Y" is a judgment made with respect to something. A rich person may well be worse off than a poor person with respect to health, and that seems a (defeasible) reason for extending the richer person extra resources of the kind for which she has the greater need. Although it may be the case that we should restructure the health care system overall so as to benefit those who are worse off with respect to their general social and economic standing, trade-offs regarding specific scarce goods within a health care system could still be appropriately influenced by worst-off-with-respect-to-health considerations. What this might require on the part of those engaged in such allocation decisions is the conviction that the system as a whole was in general "just enough" to serve as a sphere whose particular goods could be allocated as a particular kind.

But the particular difficulty in the case of Ms. Functional and Mr. Close-Knit is that we face a situation in which Mr. Close-Knit's health status is a function of his family relationships. It is due to them that he is better off, and, on the view being discussed here, it would seem that we should calculate his status counterfactually: How poorly off would he be without the irrelevant factor of his family's support? Otherwise, it would seem that the family's contribution is being dismissed as an invisible, costless resource, perhaps on par with whatever amount of physical or psychological reserve against disease anyone might have as a result of their own constitution. However, it might be argued that Mr. Close-Knit is, in fact, better off than Ms. Functional and that withdrawing the supportive care necessary for maintaining his relative advantage is no more justifiable than would be a family's actively trying to further traumatize a relative, were that a likely way of increasing his chances to receive scarce care.[24]

Coping with the Indeterminacy in the Worst-Off Principle

Neither the theory-based nor the intuitive criticisms discussed here demonstrate that we should set allocation policies in ways indifferent to the question of the appropriate degree of priority for the worst off. But neither is it clear what priority the worst off can justly claim.

One problem is determining how to balance the worst-off principle with other morally relevant constraints and goals that we encounter in thinking about allocation. Imagine three cases:

1. Jack and Jill are both candidates to be the last new patient that a highly talented clinician can admit to her caseload. Other available helping professionals are less skilled in responding successfully to the problem they share. Jack is slightly worse off than Jill. Jill, however, would gain much more than Jack from interacting with this therapist.[25]
2. In this scenario, Jack is still slightly worse off, but Jill would gain only moderately more than Jack.
3. Now, Jill's gain over the slightly worse-off Jack would be only marginal.

Many variations are possible, of course, and many responses might seem reasonable. In the initial case, many might think that best outcome considerations should be determinative; in the second case, that Jill's advantage in terms of outcome and Jack's advantage in terms of need should balance each other out, and the therapist should choose randomly, giving each a fair chance; in the final case, that Jack's being worse off should take precedence over Jill's marginal advantage.

In such situations, we typically rely on our sense of what Michael Stocker has called "normative gaps";[26] if the difference in relative benefit between Jack and Jill is "big enough," we will reverse any initial presumption in favor of the worst off, for example. This raises the question of whether we can be directed by principle or must rely on judgment to assess the size and significance of the gaps. How much extra benefit with what degree of probability must Jill expect from therapy if her claim is to be preferred to the slightly worse-off Jack?

Although there may be intuitively clear cases, theoretical illumination often gives out, and the decision rests with the perception. What the discussion thus far would indicate is that worst-off considerations are pertinent, that such considerations can be focused on certain kinds of comparisons and need not be global, and that there is no good reason to think them determinative in general.

Case Discussion

I have attempted to make reasonable the following views: theoretical challenges to the appropriateness of special attention to the worst off do not clearly succeed; intuitive difficulties with the principle can be parried; the principle can be given a scope that is limited so as to be useful in a way that is not outrageously arbitrary. I have also suggested that attention to the principle could illuminate but not always determine judgment in "fine-grained" allocation decisions. I now want to test that claim by considering cases introduced into the literature by James Sabin in collaboration with Normal Daniels.[27]

The Case of HG

Imagine a prepaid HMO that serves 350,000 people. Clinicians are salaried and there are a fixed population, budget, and resources. The strains of balancing these resources fall on the physician, because there is no third-party review. Clinicians have 14.5 direct clinical hours per week and are expected over the course of a year to take on forty-six new patients.

HG is a midlife caregiver who works with the disabled and who is a member of an ethnic minority. He has a family history of alcoholism but is not himself a substance abuser. Mr. G is reasonably effective in his work, has many friends, but has no enduring, intimate relationships. Prozac and focal psychotherapy for six to eight hours over the course of ten appointments has lifted his depression and returned him to baseline. However, HG believes that he is capable of making significant improvements in his life and, accordingly, requests to meet with his therapist for a half-hour every two weeks. The clinician agrees that further gains are possible.

Mr. G. seems a highly functional person. He does important work fairly well, and he enjoys several important human relationships. He seems to be a paradigm of someone who, while being a real candidate for treatment, is not likely to make very large relative gains and not likely to fare well in competition for the scarce resource of therapist time if the therapist is inclined to be guided by a policy of maximizing relative gain. Even if the therapist is sensitive to worst-off considerations, there may seem to be no reason not to concur with this assessment. The appropriate judgment would seem to be to allow Mr. G access to the time just in case and to the extent that no one worse off or likelier to benefit more is presented for therapy.

However, under the guidance of a better articulated understanding of the worst-off principle, the therapist might reason as follows. Mr. G has never been able to form lasting intimate relationships; this is not a trivial loss. Further, he has worked below capacity all his adult life—perhaps twenty-five years now. Given these considerations, he can reasonably be seen as quite poorly off in terms of the dimension of need. Although care is not a matter of urgency to him, the course of his life as a whole, its success or failure overall, may hinge on his ability to relate better to people and to work more effectively. It seems in the light of these considerations that Mr. G's therapist should extend the extra sessions to him, on the understanding that they may have to be interrupted, postponed, or even terminated should clearly worse-off candidates for treatment appear. However, in assessing the defensibility of interrupting the extra sessions, the therapist should consider not only the urgency of those who present more dramatic problems but their neediness. This might be a case in which Mr. G's age might support him against younger candidates.

The Case of PW

Ms. W began experiencing paranoia in her early twenties. She has done poorly when hospitalized and is marginally functional, only able to hold onto jobs that are very clearly defined. When her illness surfaced again, it took the form of delusional preoccupation with her disease. PW has consistently refused medication and has experienced only marginal improvements over the past two and a half years. PW wants to continue appointments although her doctors anticipate only minor improvement without the use of medication.

Consider PW's case with an eye to seeing how someone persuaded of the importance of the worst-off principle might deliberate. Ms. W is clearly badly off, but is she badly off with respect to the kind of therapy she is willing to accept? Perhaps given the small improvement that can reasonably be expected from talk therapy, she is not badly off with respect to its being withheld, as it would do little to ameliorate her condition.

Contrast Ms. W's case with that of an end-stage cardiac patient, Ms. Y, who is expected to die soon without a transplant. She is surely worse off than Mr. A, whose end-stage cardiac disease is less advanced but is also suffering from a kidney stone. However, suppose the rare resource in the system is not just transplantable hearts but also morphine. Ms. Y, although uncomfortable, is not in the kind of severe pain that Mr. A is facing. Should the fact that she is worse off overall mean that she gets the morphine? Will giving it to Mr. A make someone who is already better off, better off still? That would only seem to be the case if our lives lack distinct dimensions of assessment. Mr. A is surely better off than Ms. Y with respect to the concerns that prompt cardiac transplantation—his situation is not as urgent—but not with respect to the concerns that prompt administering morphine.

Analogously, we might wish to argue that Mr. G has a claim to the extra therapeutic time, because it is a good with respect to which he is worse off for the lack of than is Ms. W. If, on the other hand, Ms. W were to accept medication and thus enhance the potential effectiveness of talk therapy, such therapy might well become a resource whose lack would be an explanation of her being poorly off and hence something she would need.

The Case of the DPs

The DPs are the devoted parents of a twenty-year-old schizophrenic daughter. They have worked hard to provide a tolerant, stable, and consistent environment for her. Unfortunately, a change in her medications was poorly tolerated, and the daughter wound up in the hospital. After nine days, the daughter was ready to be discharged. However, the DPs asked if she could be discharged after the weekend, as they had made important plans which, as their daughter's caregivers, they otherwise had no opportunity to carry out.

In this case, the argument for extending the extra hospital time would seem to be along the following lines. The DPs' care is a crucial therapeutic resource for the patient. The senses in which she is badly off include her need for just the resources that her parents can provide. In giving her the extra hospital time, the system is in effect allocating funds to ensure the continued viability of an essential therapeutic resource. Utilization Review is not at all likely to look at the matter in this fashion. Could the daughter's physician morally defend authorizing the extra time, despite the concerns of utilization reviewers?

Physicians sometimes make allocation decisions as investments. For example, as fetal heart sounds cannot be heard in an anxious pregnant woman who is prone to present frequently to the emergency room, a physician might judge that an ultrasound is indicated, not because it would affect therapeutic decision making, but because reassurance might keep her out of the emergency room. If such investments are ever warranted, it is perhaps worth considering making one in this case. The difficulty in turning to preference for the worst off for determining how that consideration should turn out is that it is hard to know just over whom this patient is enjoying preference. In expending resources for hospital days for the DPs' daughter, the physicians are making a limited contribution to the family's resilience and hence increasing the chance (so one assumes) that the parents will be able to continue to care for their daughter in the home. If the resource that is scarce is hospital beds, and someone worse off than the daughter is being denied access because she's taking it up, it would seem that preference for the worst off would direct that the parents' request not be honored. There is nothing obviously counterintuitive about this result.

Preference for the worst off is a principle that stems from powerful moral intuitions. It is, however, an internally complex notion whose diverse dimensions appropriately call for attention in making allocation decisions. These added complexities may counter any hope we may have cherished that just systems of allocating scarce resources would have clear, powerful, and largely determinative constraints; indeed, unpacking their internal complexities and setting them into balance with other morally relevant dimensions may make the process of just allocation messier, less efficient, more contestable, less amenable to algorithm, and more reliant on judgment. It is also possible that it should make it, at the same time, morally more defensible.

Notes

1. The way I set up and pursue this topic is heavily indebted to Frances Kamm's work, both in *Morality, Mortality, vol. 1: Death and Whom to Save from It* (New York: Oxford, 1993), and in her contributions to The Hastings Center project, which gives rise to the present volume. That in large part she constructed the framework has no connection, of course, to any clumsiness I may display in moving within it.

2. John Rawls, *A Theory of Justice* (Cambridge, Mass.: Harvard University Press, 1971). See, for example, his discussions in chapter 2, in particular sections 10 and 16.

3. Kamm, *Morality, Mortality*.

4. Amartya Sen, *On Economic Inequality* (Oxford: Oxford University Press, 1973).

5. Aristotle *Politics* 1282b18.

6. Dan Brock, "Priority to the Worse Off in Health-Care Resource Prioritization," in *Medicine and Social Justice: Essays on the Distribution of Health Care*, ed. Rosamond Rhodes, Margaret P. Battin, and Anita Silvers (Oxford: Oxford University Press, 2002), 362–72.

7. See Frances Kamm, "Whether to Discontinue Nonfutile Use of a Scarce Resource," chapter 3 of this book.

8. Rawls, *A Theory of Justice*, 27.

9. Bernard Williams, "A Critique of Utilitarianism," in *Utilitarianism: For and Against*, ed. J. J. C. Smart and Bernard Williams (Cambridge: Cambridge University Press, 1973), 116.

10. Williams, "A Critique of Utilitarianism," 117.

11. Cheshire Calhoun's fascinating paper "Standing for Something," *Journal of Philosophy* 92 (May 1995): 235–60, argues strongly that Williams's analysis of integrity is defective, and, in any case, that deontological systems could be just as much enemies of his sense of integrity as are consequentialist systems. But, for my purposes, these are not serious problems. As Calhoun sees it, the difficulty with Williams's analysis is that he misidentifies integrity with "the conditions for continuing as the same self." Further, the havoc utilitarianism plays with integrity (in the Williams sense) seems actually to be a matter of the uncompromising impartiality of some moral systems, including deontology. But rupturing the conditions for "continuing as the same self" seems to me a worrisome matter, even if it is not identical with attacking integrity. And, if that insistence on rigorous impartiality is relaxed, there is in principle room for the persistence of selves and for moral norms, such as the worst-off principle, as well—but none for utilitarianism.

12. Jonathan Dancy, "A Particularist's Progress," in *Moral Particularism*, ed. Brian Hooker and Margaret Little (Oxford: Oxford University Press, 2002), 132.

13. In addition to the concerns of Cheshire Calhoun discussed in note 11, see Derek Parfit's reflections on the ontology of selves in, for example, his "Later Selves and Moral Principles," in *Philosophy and Personal Relations*, ed. Alan Montifiore (Montreal, Canada: McGill-Queens University Press, 1973), as well as in his *Reasons and Persons* (Oxford: Oxford University Press, 1984).

14. See Eric Rakowski, "The Just Allocation of Mental Health Care," chapter 4 of this book.

15. See Rawls's discussion of these conditions in section 26 of *A Theory of Justice*.

16. Rawls, *A Theory of Justice*, 155.

17. R. C. Kessler et al., "A Methodology for Estimating the 12-Month Prevalence of Serious Mental Illness," in *Mental Health, United States, 1999*, ed R. W. Manderscheid and M. J. Henderson (Rockville, Md.: Center for Mental Health Services, 1999), 99–109.

18. See Derek Parfit's discussion of continuity, identity, and "what matters" in *Reasons and Persons* (Oxford: Oxford University Press, 1984).

19. See, for discussion, Howard H. Goldman, Richard G. Frank, and Martin S. Gaynor, "What Level of Government? Balancing the Interests of the State and the Local Community," in *What Price Mental Health? The Ethics and Politics of Setting Priorities*, ed. Philip J. Boyle and Daniel Callahan (Washington, D.C.: Georgetown University Press, 1995), 208–15.

20. See Kamm, *Morality, Mortality*, 234ff.

21. See Kamm, *Morality, Mortality*, chap. 12.

22. Kamm alludes to Michael Walzer's *Spheres of Justice* (New York: Basic, 1983) on p. 108 of *Morality, Mortality*.

23. For further critical discussion, see James Lindemann Nelson, "Measured Fairness, Situated Justice: Feminist Reflections on Health Care Rationing," *Kennedy Institute of Ethics Journal* 6, no. 1 (1996): 53–68.

24. Compare this case with a variant in which it is a medical intervention that accounts for Mr. Close-Knit's better off status vis-à-vis Ms. Functional, and it is his professional caregivers who threaten to withdraw it so that he will decompensate to a level comparable to hers.

25. I assume that the qualitatively distinct benefit of normality, as discussed earlier, is not available for Jill.

26. In Michael Stocker, *Plural and Conflicting Values* (Oxford: Clarendon Press, 1990).

27. James E. Sabin and Norman Daniels, "Determining 'Medical Necessity' in Mental Health Practice," *Hastings Center Report* 24, no.6 (1994): 5,13.

CHAPTER 10

Ethical Issues for Providers, Patients, and Managers

Tia Powell

THE SHIFT FROM fee-for-service to managed care has substantially changed the activities of the three major participants in health care: providers, patients, and payers. As the nature of participation in health care changes, new ethical obligations arise from these changing activities. Although corporations and patients face new ethical challenges, this chapter focuses primarily on obligations for health care providers. Specifically, physicians within managed care face three new ethical obligations: to collaborate fully when accepting patients under a plan, to appeal when benefit decisions controvert medical judgment, and to evaluate ethical and clinical standards of managed care entities. None of these ethical obligations is easy to meet. However, it is in the effort to meet these challenges that physicians can maintain ethical standards within the evolving domain of managed care.

Specific clinical examples will come from the field of mental health. Issues of the stigma of illness, fluctuating decisional capacity, and confidentiality all affect psychiatric patients differently than they do general medical patients. These differences suggest a particular need for a continuing examination of the ethical implications of managed care within the domain of mental health.[1]

Perhaps the most essential feature of managed care is the change from decisions made exclusively by individual practitioners and patients to decisions in which a managed care organization has some role in terms of oversight and/or treatment planning. The degree of participation varies widely, of course, but all managed care companies do enter into this formerly private realm to some degree. Both benefits and liabilities derive from this change; benefits include greater standardization, which may decrease idiosyncratic, wasteful, or harmful care, whereas potential liabilities accrue from the loss of privacy, lack of flexibility in individual cases, and the subversion of clinical goals to economic ones.

As we assess new health care systems, we will repeatedly confront the question of how to balance cost containment against quality of care. This problem leads us directly to the issue of who will make treatment decisions, and on what basis. In theory, managed care decisions ought to follow from appropriate collaborations between patients, clinicians, and payers. As opponents of managed care quickly point out, practice does not always coincide with theory. The heart of the problem, then, is to design such collaborations to ensure an ethically appropriate balance of power between the various parties, with their sometimes conflicting interests.

Keeping an Eye on the Invisible Hand

Perhaps, one might argue, we need not worry about how to balance the competing interests of patients, providers, and payers. Managed care entities that do not satisfy will simply not survive; the problem will take care of itself. This viewpoint that the market will drive out those managed mental health care companies whose product is substandard has many flaws, particularly when applied to the delivery of health care. The market will indeed select winners and losers, but not by the only possible criterion and not necessarily by the best one. Profitable companies survive; profit, however, bears only a tangential relationship to quality. Certainly profitability may follow from efforts to create the best possible product. However, successful marketing, attractive superficial features, and cheaply constructed products may all enhance profit without reflecting quality. This problem is particularly acute in health care, where some aspects of quality are hard for consumers to evaluate. For instance, consumers can readily judge features such as an attractive hospital environment and good food, but the rates of complications for a particular surgeon or a particular surgery are not apparent unless someone else gathers the data and makes it accessible to the patient. However, although an attractive environment is not unimportant, the chances of surviving cardiac surgery with a minimum of complications is an issue of more lasting significance in evaluating the quality of health care. This example is not a fictitious one. Managed care companies in Los Angeles and Rochester, New York, chose cheaper institutions to provide coronary artery bypass graft (CABG) surgery for their patients—despite significantly higher mortality rates for the procedure at those institutions relative to their competitors.[2] Perhaps it is examples such as these that cause Eli Ginzberg and others to caution against the belief that markets will reform health care, where government has failed.[3] From an ethics viewpoint, a reliance on market factors alone does not provide a sufficiently equitable way to balance the interests of patients, payers, and providers.

The following case offers another disturbing example of how economic and other factors winnow out managed care companies. The conflict here reveals a denigration of clinical standards relative to economic goals. In this instance, a large behavioral care corporation took on the mental health care of the employees of the state of Ohio.[4] An audit after two years revealed numerous instances of inadequate care, such as offering only two sessions to a young woman diagnosed with major depression. Further, the managed care company claimed it would spend 9 of 14 million dollars allotted over two years on direct patient care. Auditors discovered that less than half that sum went to treatment, with the rest going to overhead and profits. Appropriately, the state did not renew the company's contract. However, the next contract went not to a company that proposed better quality assurance or significant alterations in the way treatment decisions were made but to one that guaranteed radically cheaper treatment.

This example, though not representative of all managed care, is an important one for various reasons. First, as powerful an entity as the state of Ohio apparently purchased behavioral health care that lacked minimally acceptable treatment standards and quality control. Purchasers with less clout are unlikely to fare better in negotiating terms for their employees. Second, untreated mental illness leads to significant morbidity and mortality.

When the purchaser, not the managed care entity, performed its audit, poor care was uncovered. However, in those two years, Ohio's employees would have suffered not only significant disability and a large number of lost work days but also a number of preventable deaths. Unless the quality of treatment improves with the new, vastly cheaper mental health care company, these workers may face the same degree of suffering over the next two years. And they will continue to suffer, and some to die, until there is a system in place that looks not only to cost but also to quality.

Some advocates of managed care dismiss the notion that cost controls lead to lesser quality. Rather, these proponents of managed care assert that cost controls can simultaneously improve quality while decreasing costs. Many mental health professionals disagree with this assertion and are enraged by it. Professional organization newsletters are still full of articles about outrageous practices by managed care entities around the country. Nonetheless, some organizations in the early years of managed care (i.e., the late 1980s and early 1990s) did in fact manage to achieve improved quality and lower cost. For instance, managed care pushed practitioners to avoid hospitalization when adequate outpatient treatment was available, often with the outcome of better and less restrictive treatment for patients.[5] However, additional cost cuts that improve quality may be hard to come by. Respected researchers such as Kenneth Wells are skeptical of the claim that costs can continually decline without sacrificing quality.[6] Through his work on the Medical Outcomes Study (MOS), Wells reaches the conclusion that well-designed managed mental health care may increase value, that is, what you get for what you pay. However, improved quality tends to increase costs rather than decrease them. Thus excellent mental health care can exist within a context of respect for resource allocation, but cost cuts must be balanced against clinical considerations.[7]

A New Ethical Obligation: Cooperation

As Victor Fuchs noted in his presidential address to the American Economics Association, "One of the greatest errors of health policy-makers today is their assumption that market competition or government regulation are the only instruments available to control health care."[8] One of the forces that Fuchs stresses is professional integrity. He makes a cogent argument that the goals of health care reform cannot be met unless careful attention is paid to the protection of professional standards in medicine.

Some leaders in the field of psychiatry have suggested that it is not possible to maintain professional integrity within the managed care context.[9] They argue that psychiatrists should refuse to participate in managed care. However, such a move is unethical, for it would leave vast numbers of our already poorly served patients with even fewer options. This chapter rejects the notion that ethical physicians ought to avoid managed care entirely. In addition to being unethical, such a stance is no longer compatible with the psychiatrist's economic survival. Numerous studies document the radical increase in the percent of patients treated within the context of managed care, as opposed to fee-for-service medicine.[10] Neither does this chapter support the practice of participating in a manner calculated to subvert the process. Rather, mental health providers have an ethical obligation to cooperate fully when they agree to treat patients within the context of managed care.

A number of implications follow from this ethical obligation of cooperation with managed care. Rather than viewing interactions with managed care entities as categorically wrong intrusions into the doctor-patient dyad, physicians who treat managed care patients need to view themselves and their expertise in a new context. Health care providers are part of a team, not soloists, and need to develop effective communication skills in order to secure appropriate treatment for their patients. Negotiation, not command, is the appropriate modality for team members to use with one another.

A number of writers argue convincingly that the definition and understanding of professionalism need to change to reflect current realities. David Rothman, for instance, scoffs at the notion that managed care has for the first time introduced economic factors as a new and deleterious influence on medical professionalism.[11] David Mechanic offers a cogent analysis of ways in which medical professionalism needs to adapt to the current practice of medicine.[12] He condemns the practice of teaching medical students and residents to cheat managed care entities and to undermine the system whenever possible. Rather, he hopes physicians will focus on teaching trainees to retain their role as the patient's advocate. An increased emphasis on communication and negotiation skills might further this end.

One way to shore up professional standards and assert the rightful place of clinical wisdom in treatment decisions is to emphasize the role of treatment guidelines in managed mental health care. Treatment guidelines must be drafted with due respect for scientific knowledge about mental conditions and their treatment. Sifting through quantities of research data and limiting the influence of financial, political, and other influences is no small matter in this task.[13] Although the creation of treatment guidelines is complex in any field, the task is especially difficult in mental health care, because of the factionalism among different mental health providers who may stand to gain if one treatment is touted as superior to another. The need for scientifically valid guidelines is therefore all the greater in mental health. Happily, there has been an explosion of research in recent years in the area of evidence-based practice in psychiatry, as well as in other fields. Websites, conferences, journals, and professional organization treatment guidelines all contribute valuable information to this process.[14]

Managed care plans must also recognize the capacity of providers to individualize treatments in ways that guidelines cannot. Plans that discourage input either in the formation of guidelines or in the attempts to appropriately modify them in the service of individual patients cannot expect a spirit of cooperation from providers. A plan that prevents adequate input from clinicians will not provide high-quality care. Those plans that stress efficacy and solid outcomes research, with the ability to revise guidelines as knowledge advances, will offer the best care without compromising physician integrity.

A mental health care provider who wishes to adhere to the obligation to cooperate would need to do so at a number of different levels within the system. As a new managed care entity forms, the ethical practitioner would want to help form the standards of care, determining, for instance, which illnesses are covered and what sorts of treatments are reimbursed. The cooperative practitioner would want to guarantee that these plans and limits are all solidly based on best clinical practices. Next, the cooperative practitioner would wish to communicate clearly to patients all available treatment options. If an appropriate option is not covered under the plan, the ethically cooperative practitioner would need to advocate that the patient should receive such treatment. Of course, in order for the health care provider to adhere to these requirements, he or she must be working within an ethical organization. Clearly, not all managed care entities meet these standards. Thus in order to meet the ethical duty to cooperate, the provider must also face the ethical duty to evaluate the standards of the managed care organization.

Appeals Processes

The shift to managed care is a shift from a two-part (doctor-patient) decision-making team to a three-part (doctor-patient-payer) team. The payer is inherently at risk for overemphasizing issues of cost, and thus appropriate counterbalancing influences should come from doctors and patients. Health care providers can buttress their point of view with well-researched treatment guidelines. When individual patients' needs do not coincide with standard recommendations, providers can offer reasoned arguments and clinical data as they request exceptions. Indeed, both legal precedent and ethical standards support the physician's duty to appeal in such cases.[15] The American Medical Association's published guidelines address, among other issues, the physician's duty to act as an advocate for patients within managed care.[16] However, data and argument are ineffective when managed care entities have no true appeals process.

In the initial years of managed care, appeals processes varied widely among different organizations. Some entities had virtually no appeals process. In these companies, arguments began and ended with a utilization reviewer aggressively stating that the service was not "medically necessary" and would not be covered. Other organizations, particularly those with a longer history, had rigorous appeals processes with consumer participation and various levels of review. Still other organizations appeared to have one (usually admirable) policy on paper, while radically departing from this process in actual practice. In response to this disarray within the industry, various professional bodies drew up recommendations for appeals processes, and a presidential commission was charged to propose policies for appeals. Thus, in 1997, the President's Advisory Commission on Consumer Protection and Quality in the Health Care Industry made public its set of recommendations for dispute resolution.[17] Over the last several years, mechanisms for dispute resolution have evolved dramatically. At this point, all states require health plans to have appeals processes as a condition of licensure.[18]

However, appeals processes remain imperfect, particularly as applied to mental health care. Even in organizations that only supply mental health care, the medical director need not be a psychiatrist. Some plans only infrequently call upon a psychiatrist to assess appeals. When such expert advice is requested, the psychiatrist is hired as a consultant on a case-by-case basis. Conflicts of interest abound in this arrangement, for consultants who wish to be rehired might do well to side with the company. The appeals system is generally not described in the literature used to recruit physicians. Neither do companies disclose data on the percent of cases appealed or on the percent of decisions changed by appeal. Thus, clinicians who wish to evaluate the ethical soundness of a managed care organization before joining will not succeed in doing so on the basis of solid information, but must rely on rumor and general impressions.

A covert but powerful force inhibiting appeals is that they require considerable uncompensated physician time and effort. Assertions that payment for appeals is included in the basic physician fee are disingenuous, as such fees represent ever decreasing amounts and are described as compensation for clinical visits of ever shorter duration. Physicians now required to see patients in fifteen-minute or briefer intervals, regardless of the complexity of the case, for a substantially reduced fee, are not likely to view the appeals process as an activity for which they are compensated. The most radically pro-physician and anti-business solution to this problem would be to reward physicians who successfully appeal cases. Although highly improbable, I cite such a theoretical possibility to highlight the fact that physicians who appeal cases now are essentially never rewarded but only punished, either through the loss of large amounts of uncompensated time or by actually being dismissed from managed care organizations. Physicians have an ethical obligation to appeal inappropriate decisions. Because such efforts are thus consistent with the highest standards of professional integrity, it is disturbing that the current system significantly inhibits such activity.

Different types of managed care models may affect the provider's capacity to appeal in different ways. In a staff model organization, the provider works only for the single corporate entity and receives a salary that may actually include time for administrative work. Efforts to appeal decisions might allow the provider to push for a change in treatment guidelines, a change from which the provider would benefit through greater work satisfaction and a sense of professional integrity. On the other hand, too much effort in the direction of appealing decisions or changing established guidelines might label the provider as a troublemaker. This label is more ominous when it comes from one's sole employer than when it comes from a payer who provides only a small percent of income. Thus, the physician employed by a staff model organization faces both great potential punishments and great potential rewards as a result of actively appealing treatment decisions.

By contrast, in the network model the provider is not a salaried employee of the managed care organization, but rather is paid according to the number of patients or treatments provided. Physicians may belong to many such networks simultaneously, depending on the area of the country or the practitioner's specialty. Appeals for this provider are quite different from that of the staff model employee. The provider may not have any previous relationship or prospect of a continued relationship with the other parties in the appeals process. Rather, the managed care reviewer may be to the provider only a disembodied voice, anonymous and geographically distant from both clinician and patient. If the provider has a wide choice of managed care companies with which to do business, either because of a successful practice or a diversified market, the wise choice may be to decline further business with an organization whose decisions demand appeal. The provider will benefit only modestly from appealing any given decision, for this company supplies only a percentage of the provider's patients. Further, because the provider is paid only for clinical work and not for administrative efforts, the appeals process is likely to cost more in terms of lost clinical time. On the other hand, the provider has less to fear from this single organization than would be the case for a staff model employee. Thus different models of managed care impose different ethical challenges on mental health and other providers. In any case, improved treatment guidelines and greater support for appeals processes are necessary ingredients for ethical managed mental health care.

Evaluation

The third ethical obligation generated by the emerging system of managed care is the duty to evaluate the ethical and clinical standards of companies with which the clinician works. This evaluation is not done once and then completed, but it is an ongoing process that continues as long as the association does. In part, the clinician reviews whether or not the organization's structure promotes or inhibits the possibility of meeting the obligations to cooperate and to appeal. If an organization is designed so that a clinician cannot meet ethical obligations within it, the provider must change the organization or leave it. One cannot ethically remain in association with a managed care organization that offers unacceptable levels of care, that does not respond to efforts to change inappropriate guidelines and practices, and that does not provide a sufficient appeals process.

Daniels and Sabin, in a much-quoted article, outlined four conditions for fairness in allocating health care resources.[19] Those managed care entities that promote these conditions operate in an ethical context. The four requirements are (1) an accessible rationale for treatment limitations, (2) clear evidence that this treatment plan promotes the health of individuals and groups within the system, (3) a robust dispute resolution system, and (4) adequate mechanisms to guarantee adherence to the first three conditions. Thus in order for a health care provider to meet the obligation to cooperate, he or she must be working within an ethical context, as defined earlier.

Unfortunately, a physician is not likely to find all of the information needed to evaluate a company in advance of employment. Some information that is available to consumers, in the form of "report cards" for managed care companies, will assist providers in their evaluation. However, companies may not supply other types of useful information, such as the process by which treatment guidelines are determined or appeals adjudicated. Again, this ethical obligation to evaluate exists, but the system as currently structured imposes barriers to clinicians who wish to meet it.

The evaluation of the organization's ethical standards must also include an assessment of standards of disclosure to patients, for the degree of disclosure of relevant benefit and treatment information to patients is a measure of the organization's respect for patient autonomy. Indeed, issues of disclosure have figured largely in some of the most acrimonious exchanges between physicians and plan managers. For instance, there was no ethical justification for the "gag clauses" contained in some early managed care contracts. These clauses forbid doctors to discuss a number of issues with patients, including the option of pursuing effective treatments not covered by the plan. Physicians must not only be permitted but encouraged to discuss various treatment options with patients, even those treatments not covered but that are potentially beneficial. If physicians have ethical obligations to appeal denials of care, they are equally compelled to discuss such appeals with patients. Exclusion of the patient from the decision-making process is exactly the sort of erosion of autonomy that an ethical system must avoid. However, the outcry from the public against gag clauses was so great that they may be viewed as managed care's greatest gift to its opponents.[20] Managed care advocates initially seemed peculiarly insensitive to the public reaction, thus fueling the flames of a violent backlash. For instance, Mark Jordan, a lawyer for Kaiser Permanente, was quoted in the *New York Times* as saying, "Why should a managed care physician be required to advertise that he or she might reduce services to increase income?"[21] The reaction to such comments led to major changes in the industry's stance. Between voluntary changes and legislative efforts, the gag clause has essentially disappeared.

An important area for ethical evaluation is the method of compensation for providers. Because such agreements potentially contain conflicts of interest, patients should know about them. However, simply informing patients of such contractual agreements is not sufficient. The language of contracts is notoriously obscure to the average reader, let alone to the average sick person. In an interesting review of patients' understanding of physician financial incentives, Tracy Miller finds that few patients comprehend the implications of different plans unless they are offered significant educational opportunities.[22] Thus simply stating the facts about physician compensation does not lead to full information for the patient. An additional objection to mere disclosure is that many patients have limited freedom to leave a plan with poor provisions, either because choice is controlled by employers or because of preexisting illness.

Finally, contracts that base large amounts of the physician's pay on his or her ability to decrease costs can be damaging to medical decision making, whether patients know about them or not. When large percentages of a doctor's income depend on the ability to contain costs, patients may begin to wonder about the doctor's motivation. For example, a patient may wonder if surgery is no longer recommended because the doctor is nearing a budgetary limit or because it is no longer in the patient's best interest. Industry representatives wish to maintain the freedom to compensate doctors for withholding care, because that latitude may help the company survive in a competitive environment. This approach does not reveal appropriate concern for the need to protect patients from excessive cost cutting. Rather, it focuses on the organization's need to survive, even if quality suffers. Not surprisingly, some groups have called for states to increase monitoring requirements for managed care and to include in such monitoring an assessment of "risk arrangements and their impact on access and quality of care."[23]

Unfortunately for advocates of ethical managed care, the Supreme Court dealt a blow to efforts to limit unjust compensation schemes. The case of *Pegram v. Herdrich* is illustrative in a number of ways.[24] Mrs. Herdrich received medical care from a physician-owned HMO. She complained to Dr. Lori Pegram about abdominal pain, but no workup was done on the first visit. The patient returned six days later, when Dr. Pegram noted a large, inflamed abdominal mass. She ordered an ultrasound for eight days later, at a distant facility owned by her HMO. Mrs. Herdrich's inflamed appendix ruptured before the ultrasound, however, causing her serious complications and a prolonged hospital stay. (Ironically, the diagnosis of acute appendicitis might well have been determined via the cost-effective means of a thorough physical exam.) Mrs. Herdrich was particularly enraged when she learned that Dr. Pegram received a year-end bonus based on savings from reduced expenditures on patient care. The patient won her state malpractice claim, but her claim that the clinic breached its fiduciary duty went all the way to the U.S. Supreme Court, where it was struck down. The unanimous decision stressed that Congress wished to support cost containment in health care and that the Court could see no reason to involve itself in HMOs' efforts to compensate doctors for doing just that. Thus we cannot hope that in the immediate future we will see an end to all compensation schemes of dubious ethical validity.

Advocates of ethical managed health care describe more just systems of compensation. James Sabin, for instance, proposes that compensation mirror efforts to meet performance standards.[25] When Massachusetts contracted for Medicaid mental health services, it designed the contract so that compensation increased with better performance, not because of withholding funds budgeted for services.

Currently there is an uneasy tension between efforts to curtail unethical policies within managed care and the effort to inform patients about the policies and let them draw their own conclusions. To understand this tension, a useful analogy may be made between the health care and securities industries. In the financial world, the question of how best to protect individual investors has generated vigorous debate since the 1930s. There are advocates for disclosure who feel that once investors have information, it is their responsibility to assess it and act wisely. Opponents argue that wily institutions may use excessively technical language that investors cannot comprehend. Therefore there is no real disclosure. Still other factions insist that even effective disclosure is not enough; limits must be established as to what offers can be made to the unwary.

If we compare the example of the securities industry to that of medicine, we find similarities and differences. The factions within the debate are similar. Managed care organizations tend to argue that contracts with disclosure protect consumers adequately. Consumers do not always agree and may advocate for better efforts at disclosure, as well as limits to acceptable policies. However, a model that relies on disclosure alone to protect patients is not appropriate in medicine, and less so in psychiatry than in other branches of medicine. For instance, denial of illness is extremely common for many psychiatric patients, including those suffering from substance abuse, eating disorders, and schizophrenia. It is not protective of such patients to suggest that they examine insurance policies to see if benefits are appropriate to their needs, when their very illness may prevent them from adequately assessing their needs. Furthermore, decision-making capacity can erode as psychiatric symptoms increase, making a reliance on disclosure alone problematic.

In addition, the extraordinary stigma of psychiatric illness can inhibit psychiatric patients from revealing their health care needs, no matter how acutely they may understand them. Patients are not adequately protected when they are simply informed of the rules of a system that contains conflicts of interest and ethical lapses. Thus undue emphasis on disclosure, a technique that emphasizes the patient's autonomy, without any limits on what terms are permissible, is an inadequate protection of patients' interests. An undue emphasis on disclosure de-emphasizes the obligation for mental health professionals and managers to act responsibly and with integrity. As Ezekiel Emanuel has observed, disclosure is a necessary but not sufficient condition for ethically appropriate care.[26]

Conclusion

Various attempts to balance the interests of patients, providers, and payers within managed care are currently under way. The relative benefits and liabilities of legislation, treatment guidelines, financial incentives, and appeals processes are current areas of study. Each of these methods has significant benefits and limitations. Certainly the least useful option is for providers, managers, and policymakers to denigrate each other's motivations and contributions to the process of redesigning mental health care. Rather, our patients, and that is to say ourselves, will best be served if each group assumes it has something valuable to learn from the other. In order to conceptualize a system that appropriately balances legitimate needs of patients, payers, and providers, we must examine not only individual aspects of decision making but the ethical context in which decisions are made. Such a context must include an examination of the duties of patients, providers, and health plan managers. This article focuses on the three new ethical duties for physicians that arise from the emerging system of managed care: cooperation, appeal, and evaluation. These three duties are not meant to reside in the realm of theory but to be used as everyday tools in providing ethically sound managed mental health care. Cynicism and efforts to subvert managed care are not viable methods of maintaining professional integrity.

Rather, clinicians should strive to know the ethical standards of the organizations with which they work. Within accepted organizations, the provider cooperates fully, working as a force to promote better care and high standards. When benefit decisions do not promote the patient's best interest, the provider pursues appeals, upholding the ethical obligation to serve as the patient's advocate.

Systems of health care delivery come and go; managed care may evolve into a wholly different form in the coming years. The task of the ethical clinician is to maintain professional integrity in a changing world.

Notes

1. Philip Boyle and Daniel Callahan, "Managed Care and Mental Health: The Ethical Issues," *Health Affairs* 14, no. 3 (fall 1995): 7–22.

2. George Anders, "Who Pays the Cost of Cut-Rate Care?" *Wall Street Journal*, Tuesday, October 15, 1996, B1.

3. Eli Ginzberg, "A Cautionary Note on Market Reforms in Health Care," *JAMA* 274, no. 20 (1995): 1633–34.

4. C. Hymowitz and E. J. Pollock, "Cost-Cutting Firms Monitor Couch Time as Therapists Fret," *Wall Street Journal*, July 13, 1995, A1.

5. James E. Sabin, "Managed Care and Health Care Reform: Comedy, Tragedy and Lessons," *Psychiatric Services* 51, no. 11 (November 2000): 1392–96.

6. Kenneth B. Wells and Roland Sturm, "Care for Depression in a Changing Environment," *Health Affairs* 14, no. 3 (fall 1995): 78–89.

7. James E. Sabin, "General Hospital Psychiatry and the Ethics of Managed Care," *General Hospital Psychiatry* 17 (1995): 293–98.

8. Victor Fuchs, "Economics, Values and Health Care Reform," *American Economic Review* 86 (March 1996): i–24.

9. See, for instance, the description of the race for the presidency of the American Psychiatric Association in 1995 in John Iglehart, "Managed Care and Mental Health," *NEJM* 334 (January 11, 1996): 131–35; William Sullivan, "What Is Left of Professionalism after Managed Care?" *Hastings Center Report* 29 (March–April 1999): 7–23.

10. M. E. Oss, *Managed Behavioral Health Market Share in the United States, 1994* (Gettysburg, Pa.: Open Minds, 1994).

11. David J. Rothman, " Medical Professionalism—Focusing on the Real Issues," *NEJM* 342, no. 17 (2000): 1284–86.

12. David Mechanic, "Managed Care and the Imperative for a New Professional Ethic," *Health Affairs* 19, no. 5 (September–October 2000): 100–111.

13. S. Woolf, "Practice Guidelines: A New Reality in Medicine; I. Recent Developments," *Archives of Internal Medicine* 150 (1990): 1811–19; S. Woolf, "Practice Guidelines II: Methods of Developing Guidelines," *Archives of Internal Medicine* 152 (1992): 946–52; S. Woolf, "Practice Guidelines III: Impact on Patient Care," *Archives of Internal Medicine* 153 (1993): 2646–55.

14. See, for instance, the American Psychiatric Association set of treatment guidelines for a variety of serious mental disorders. Also see the following journals: *Journal of Evidence-Based Medicine, Evidence-Based Health Care,* and *Evidence-Based Mental Health.*

15. See *Wickline v. California,* 192 Cal. App. 3d 160 (1986), cited in R. Geraty, R. Hendren, and C. Flaa, "Ethical Perspectives on Managed Care as It Relates to Child and Adolescent Psychiatry," *Journal of the American Academy of Child and Adolescent Psychiatry* 31, no. 3 (1992): 398–402.

16. Council on Ethical and Judicial Affairs, AMA, "Ethical Issues in Managed Care," *JAMA* 273, no. 4 (1995): 330–35.

17. Advisory Commission on Consumer Protection and Quality in the Health Care Industry, "Quality First: Better Health Care for All Americans: Final Report to the President of the United States," Appendix A: Consumer Bill of Rights and Responsibilities, 1997.

18. N. Karp and E. Wood, "Health Plan Internal Consumer Dispute Resolution Practices: Highlights from a National Study," *Journal of Health Care Law and Policy,* in press.

19. Norman Daniels and James Sabin, "Limits to Health Care: Fair Procedures, Democratic Deliberation, and the Legitimacy Problem for Insurers," *Philosophy and Public Affairs* 26, no. 4 (1997): 303–50.

20. See, for instance, the outcry when David Himmelstein was fired by, and subsequently rehired by, U.S. Healthcare for commenting on their gag clause in S. Woolhandler and D. Himmelstein, "Extreme Risk—The New Corporate Proposition for Physicians," *NEJM* 333, no. 25 (1995): 1707–08.

21. Ibid., 1707.

22. T. Miller and C. Horowitz, "Disclosing Doctors' Incentives: Will Consumers Understand and Value the Information?" *Health Affairs* 19, no. 4 (July–August 2000): 149–55.

23. Bazelon Center for Health Care Rights, "Consumer Protections," Washington, D.C.: Bazelon Center Publications, 1994), 72.

24. *Pegram v. Herdrich,* 120 S Ct 2143, 2000. Discussed in P. Appelbaum, "*Pegram v. Herdrich:* The Supreme Court Passes the Buck on Managed Care," *Psychiatric Services* 51, no.10 (2000): 1225–26.

25. James Sabin and Norman Daniels, "Public Sector Managed Behavioral Care: II. Contracting for Medicaid Services–The Massachusetts Experience," *Psychiatric Services* 50 (1999): 39–41.

26. Ezekiel Emanuel, "Medical Ethics in the Era of Managed Care: The Need for Institutional Structures Instead of Principles for Individual Cases," *Journal of Clinical Ethics* 6, no. 4 (winter 1995): 335–38.

Contributors

GARY S. BELKIN, M.D., Ph.D. is assistant professor, Harvard Medical School.

DAN W. BROCK, Ph.D., is senior scientist, Department of Clinical Bioethics, National Institutes of Health.

ALLEN E. BUCHANAN, Ph.D., is professor of public policy studies and philosophy, Duke University.

FRANCES M. KAMM, Ph.D., is Lucius Littauer Professor of Philosophy and Public Policy, Kennedy School of Government, and professor of philosophy, Department of Philosophy, Harvard University.

TERESITA MCCARTY, Ph.D., is chief of Psychiatry and Consultation Liaison Service, University of New Mexico School of Medicine.

BENTSON H. MCFARLAND, M.D., is professor of psychiatry, public health, and preventive medicine, School of Medicine, Oregon Health Sciences University.

JAMES LINDEMANN NELSON, Ph.D., is professor of philosophy and faculty associate, Center for Ethics and Humanities in the Life Sciences, Michigan State University.

DAVID A. POLLACK, M.D., is associate director, Public Psychiatry Training Program, and associate professor of psychiatry, Oregon Health Sciences University.

TIA POWELL, M.D., is a health care ethicist, National Center for Ethics in Health Care (VHA).

ERIC RAKOWSKI, D.Phil, J.D., is Edward C. Halbach Jr. Professor of Law, University of California, Berkeley.

LAURA WEISS ROBERTS, M.D., is associate director of medical student education, Department of Psychiatry, University of New Mexico School of Medicine.

SALLY K. SEVERINO, M.D., is executive vice chair, University of New Mexico School of Medicine.

Index